CHILDHOOD DISABILITY IN DEVELOPING COUNTRIES

CHILDHOOD DISABILITY IN DEVELOPING COUNTRIES

Issues in Habilitation and Special Education

Edited by

Kofi Marfo
Assistant Professor
Memorial University of Newfoundland, Canada

Sylvia Walker
Associate Professor
Howard University, Washington, D.C.

Bernard Charles
Program Officer
Carnegie Corporation of New York

PRAEGER

PRAEGER SPECIAL STUDIES • PRAEGER SCIENTIFIC

New York • Philadelphia • Eastbourne, UK
Toronto • Hong Kong • Tokyo • Sydney

Library of Congress Cataloging in Publication Data
Main entry under title:

Childhood disability in developing countries.

Includes indexes.
1. Handicapped children--Rehabilitation--Developing countries. 2. Handicapped children--Education--Developing countries. 3. Handicapped children--Developing countries--Public opinion.
I. Marfo, Kofi. II. Walker, Sylvia. III. Charles, Bernard.
RJ138.C48 1985 362.4'088054 85-20871
ISBN 0-03-007317-0

Published in 1986 by Praeger Publishers
CBS Educational and Professional Publishing, a Division of CBS Inc.
521 Fifth Avenue, New York, NY 10175 USA

6789 052 987654321

Printed in the United States of America on acid-free paper

INTERNATIONAL OFFICES

Orders from outside the United States should be sent to the appropriate address listed below. Orders from areas not listed below should be placed through CBS International Publishing, 383 Madison Ave., New York, NY 10175 USA

Australia, New Zealand
Holt Saunders, Pty, Ltd., 9 Waltham St., Artarmon, N.S.W. 2064, Sydney, Australia

Canada
Holt, Rinehart & Winston of Canada, 55 Horner Ave., Toronto, Ontario, Canada M8Z 4X6

Europe, the Middle East, & Africa
Holt Saunders, Ltd., 1 St. Anne's Road, Eastbourne, East Sussex, England BN21 3UN

Japan
Holt Saunders, Ltd., Ichibancho Central Building, 22-1 Ichibancho, 3rd Floor, Chiyodaku, Tokyo, Japan

Hong Kong, Southeast Asia
Holt Saunders Asia, Ltd., 10 Fl, Intercontinental Plaza, 94 Granville Road, Tsim Sha Tsui East, Kowloon, Hong Kong

Manuscript submissions should be sent to the Editorial Director, Praeger Publishers, 521 Fifth Avenue, New York, NY 10175 USA

Table of Contents

PREFACE

In recent years, increased attention has been given to the needs of handicapped children throughout the world. When the United Nations designated 1981 as International Year of Disabled Persons (IYDP), the event focused attention on the fact that large numbers of disabled children reside in developing countries. The United Nations Children's Fund (UNICEF) has estimated that by the year 2000 there will be over 150 million disabled children under 15 years of age in developing countries. This book represents an effort to raise awareness about the magnitude of the problem of childhood disability in developing countries and to provide some insights into how several dimensions of the problem are being addressed in different parts of the developing world.

Children in developing countries are extremely vulnerable to many biological and environmental factors which cause handicapping conditions. The principal causes of childhood disability in these countries are related to such factors as malnutrition, poor hygiene, and preventable viral and bacterial diseases that affect children and pregnant mothers. Massive preventive and community development programs embarked upon in the immediate post-independence eras have slowed down tremendously over the past few decades. The result is a sharp increase in childhood mortality and morbidity rates in many parts of the developing world. The need for improved health care, adequate nutrition, and early habilitation programs is as crucial today as it was a quarter of a century ago when most developing countries were emerging as newly independent nations.

Inspite of the advances which have been made in special education in recent years, much remains to be done if developing countries are to serve all their disabled children. In most developing countries, less than 2% of disabled persons requiring various forms of services are enrolled in educational or rehabilitation programs. Several factors impede the effective delivery of services. First, limited resources restrict all forms of services to both handicapped and nonhandicapped children. Second, difficulties in communication and transportation result in problems in developing networks and linkages between social service agencies. Third, insufficient training programs for health care, educational, and other social service personnel limit the provision of adequate services.

International efforts to provide rehabilitation services to disabled children (and adults) in the developing world have a relatively long history and have been steadily intensified in recent years. Nevertheless, prevention and community-based early habilitation are only now beginning to receive the critical attention they deserve. It is increasingly being recognized that incidence and prevalence rates far outweigh resource availability for effective provision of services; in fact, the continuing surge in incidence rates poses a serious threat to current as well as future efforts to make habilitation and rehabilitation services available to the majority of disabled persons.

The problems outlined above point to a critical need for a concerted effort by indigenous governmental and nongovernmental agencies of individual developing countries, and by international organizations, to: a) plan and implement preventive strategies aimed at a drastic reduction in the incidence of childhood disability; b) develop programs for the early habilitation of disabled children to prevent impairments from becoming handicaps; c) establish community based maternal and child care facilities and services to enhance healthy child development and upbringing; d) provide for the special educational needs of school-age disabled children in environments that would be least disruptive of normal developmental experiences; and e) work toward the development of policies, strategies, and legislative provisions which will enhance the ultimate integration of disabled children and youth into the mainstream of society.

The successful achievement of these goals rests upon a number of important first steps, including interest and research activity in the identification of various aspects of the problem—the most prevalent forms of disability; the causes of such disabilities; their distribution within the population; prospects for prevention and intervention; the nature as well as the strengths and weaknesses of existing facilities; and prospects and appropriate strategies for improving upon and/or expanding existing programs. In the 17 chapters which make up this book, authors from different parts of the world address one or more of the above issues.

The book has three parts. Part One deals with issues and research related to incidence, prevention, early detection, and habilitation. In Chapter 1, Marfo assesses the magnitude of the problem of childhood disability from an ecological perspective and discusses the 'prevention imperative' in relation to a broad range of physical-environmental as well as socio-economic and political variables that interact to nurture the problem. In Chapter 2, Fryers appraises the goals, process, and implications of screening, and provides many useful insights and suggestions for designing screening programs in developing countries. Andrada reports data on the incidence and management of cerebral palsy in Portugal in Chapter 3, and discusses current approaches to detection and early intervention in that country. In Chapter 4, Thorburn describes the development and status of early intervention programs for disabled children in four Caribbean countries: Jamaica, Barbados, Curaçao, and Haiti. Chapter 5 by Thorburn and Roeher presents a model for the preparation of rehabilitation personnel in developing countries with emphasis on Community Based Rehabilitation (CBR). In Chapter 6, Akpati presents proposals for service delivery to a neglected but sizeable population of disabled persons—those with communication disorders. In Chapter 7, Miles provides a thought-provoking analysis and critique of the planning of facilities and services for the disabled in developing countries. Part One ends with Rashid's brief data-based descriptive and evaluative report on a community-oriented physiotherapy program for children with polio in the North West Frontier Province of Pakistan.

Part Two deals with issues related to the education and training of disabled children. In Chapter 9, Baine examines the problems involved in the adoption by developing countries of assessment and curriculum materials that are based on western schedules of child development and discusses several essential elements of curriculum development for early childhood special education programs. In Chapter 10, Hughes reviews the literature on assessment of the mentally retarded and presents and describes in detail an assessment tool for use with mentally handicapped persons which he developed in Sri Lanka while serving as a consultant to the Ministry of Education in that country.

The rest of Part Two focuses on the status of special education and therapeutic services in selected parts of the developing world. Hughes examines in Chapter 11 several factors that impinge upon the development of educational services for mentally retarded children in developing countries and, in Chapter 12, Zaman describes not only the status of services for disabled children but also research efforts to ascertain the prevalence of childhood disability in Bangladesh. In Chapter 13, Walker, Marfo, Danquah, and Aidoo trace the history of special education in Ghana and provide several suggestions for improving both the quality and coverage of special education, while Csapo presents in Chapter 14 a history of the development and expansion of general as well as special education in Vietnam. Chapter 15 by Danquah is a review of the development and status of behavior therapy in developing countries.

In Part Three on social-psychological considerations, Walker examines social mores and traditional beliefs as they relate to attitudes toward the disabled in Africa. In the final chapter, Bickford and Wickham report a cross-cultural study of attitudes toward mentally retarded persons, using samples from Barbados, Canada, Kenya, Peru, Sierra Leone, and Scotland.

In preparing this book we have been guided by what we perceive to be a critical need for appropriate and relevant content in training programs which prepare various kinds of professionals (medical/nursing, rehabilitation, social work, and special education) to work in developing countries. Consequently, we hope that training institutions in developing countries as well as the hundreds of programs in Australia, Europe, and North America which train professionals for the developing world would find the book useful.

We are grateful to the contributing authors for the enthusiasm with which they responded to the call for papers, and for their continuing dedication to the objectives of the project. Our sincere appreciation goes also to several other individuals who assisted in diverse ways to make this publication possible: Jonas Darko-Yeboah and Joe Amoako-Tuffour for help with computer text processing; Thelma Anderson for clerical assistance; Myrtle Deering, Adelaide Marbell, William McDonald, Christine Baidoo, Sandra Covassi, and Rose Marfo for editorial assistance. Editorial work on the book was completed while the first editor was Coordinator of the Cognitive Education Project at the University of Alberta; we wish to thank Dr. Robert Mulcahy, the Director of the project, for his support.

We are greatly indebted to the following individuals in the United States for their generous financial support: Chester J. Trumbo, Bernard L. Charles, Joseph Giglio, and Garland Woods. Finally, we wish to thank our families for their continuing support of our efforts in the fields of rehabilitation and special education in the context of developing countries.

PART ONE: INCIDENCE, DETECTION, EARLY INTERVENTION, AND HABILITATION

1

CONFRONTING CHILDHOOD DISABILITY IN THE DEVELOPING COUNTRIES

Kofi Marfo[1]

Survey data and statistical estimates on the incidence of disability indicate that developing regions of the world account for over 70% of the world's total population of disabled persons. Evidence suggests also that many disabling conditions originate from the early developmental years (the prenatal period and the first five years of life). Although very alarming, this situation is not surprising given the welter of poverty-related hazards to which the majority of the developing world's population is exposed. This chapter examines childhood disability in relation to the quality of health care and general social welfare in developing countries.

The problem will be examined from two perspectives: childhood disability as an important issue in its own right, and as a symptomatic manifestation of models and strategies of national development that have failed to respond to the needs of the majority of the developing world's population. The second perspective, which will receive greater emphasis, will largely involve an analysis of the political, economic, and socio-cultural forces that are perpetually nurturing ecological etiologies related to childhood disability. A major thesis that will be advanced in the course of the discussion is that the hope for effectively confronting childhood disability in the developing world lies in the ability to recognize and attack the broader underlying problems of which childhood disability and its allied problems are only symptoms.

In recent years disability has frequently been defined in relation to a second terminology, *impairment*. When a loss, abnormality, or defect causes organ structure or function to deviate from generally

[1]This chapter is based on a paper presented at the 15th World Congress of Rehabilitation International, Lisbon, Portugal, June, 1984.

accepted standards—anatomically, physiologically, mentally, or psychologically—an impairment is said to exist. Disability results from impairment and refers to any limitations in or absence of ability to perform an activity or skill considered appropriate in relation to age, sex, or social-cultural norms (Wood & Bradley, 1980). In this chapter, childhood disability is defined as the existence among children of difficulties or deficiencies in ambulation, hearing, sight, speech, intellectual functioning, and social or self-help/living skills resulting from environmental deprivation or impairment to organ structure and/or function.

DEVELOPING COUNTRIES AND THE WORLD DISABILITY SITUATION

Although reliable statistical data on disabled persons in developing countries are not readily available because of limited research activity in this area, the magnitude of the problem can still be gleaned from global estimates available through international organizations and isolated country surveys usually covering one or two categories of disabilities. In 1975 it was estimated that 75% of the world's then 490 million disabled persons lived in the developing countries (Noble, 1981). By 1981 the global disabled population had risen to 514 million, and it was predicted then that by the end of the century as much as 80% of the world's disabled population would be located in the developing countries. The above estimates reveal a higher disability rate in developing countries than in the developed countries where an estimated 10% of the population are disabled. Data from several sources, including World Health Organization estimates, point to a possible 15-20% disability rate in the developing countries (Noble, 1981). To take but one example, this means that in Africa, based on 1984 population estimates, some 58 to 78 million persons are disabled. Of these some 26 to 35 million are children under 15 years of age. Given that indices of the quality of life in Africa are among the lowest in the world, the upper ends of the above ranges will likely reflect a more realistic estimate.

That disability rates are higher in the developing countries than in the technologically more advanced countries is not difficult to explain. Poverty and its social manifestations—inadequate nutrition, disease, illiteracy, inequitable distribution of social services, poor housing, poor drinking water, improper hygiene, etc.—are more prevalent in the developing than the developed countries. Indices such as average life expectancy at birth and infant and maternal mortality rates shed some light on the extent to which poverty subjects both rural and urban populations in the developing world to a quality of life that is far below an acceptable minimum standard. The sixth report on the world health situation (WHO, 1980) reveals that roughly 10% of some 122 million infants born each year will die before reaching their first birthday, and another 4% before their fifth birthday. The chances of survival are however unevenly distributed around the globe. In the technologically more advanced countries the risk of children dying before they reach adolescence is about **1** in **40** whereas in Africa the ratio is **1** in **4** and even reaches as high as **1** in **2** in some countries.

While maternal and childhood mortality rates have decreased steadily in more developed parts of the world over the past two decades, levels of mortality remain high in developing regions. In fact as Gwatkins (1979) has observed, progress in reducing infant and maternal mortality in the developing countries appears to be slowing down. Data from the World Health Organization (WHO, 1980) confirm Gwatkins' observation and point to general stagnation in the progress of development as the major cause of the slow-down. United Nations estimates for the period 1965-1969 showed that 84% of all births during that period occurred in developing countries (Djukanovic & Mach, 1975). The infant mortality rate for less developed regions of the world during that period was 140 per 1,000 live births compared to 27 per 1,000 in the technologically more advanced countries. More recent data covering the period 1970-1975 show that the slow-down in efforts to reduce mortality is very real; while the infant mortality rate for more developed regions was estimated at a range of 8 to 40 per 1,000 live births, the rate was 85 to 90 per 1,000 for Latin America, 130 per 1,000 for Northern Africa, 120-130 per 1,000 for Asia, and 200 per 1,000 for sub-Saharan Africa.

Life expectancy at birth provides a complementary picture of health status and social well-being. The lowest life expectancies among the more developed countries average 64 to 65 years for males and 70 years for females reported for countries like Portugal, USSR, Yugoslavia, and Northern Ireland. The highest expectancies are reported for Japan, Norway, and Sweden—72 to 73 years for males and 78 years for females. These figures contrast sharply with expectancies as low as 50 years in sub-Saharan Africa and between 50 and 60 years in most other developing regions of the world (see WHO, 1980).

GENERAL ENVIRONMENTAL RISKS

In developing countries the causes of childhood mortality have been more extensively and directly studied than have the causes of childhood disability, although the two conditions are strongly related. Where epidemiological studies of childhood disability have been carried out they have tended to focus on disabilities related to specific major impairments—e.g. hearing (Holborow, Martinson, & Anger, 1981) or orthopaedic impairments (Nicholas, Kratzer, Ofosu-Amaah, & Belcher, 1977; Ofosu-Amaah, Kratzer, & Nicholas, 1977; Ulfah, Parastho, Sadjimin, & Rhode, 1981). The emphasis should be made, however, that there is more to childhood disability than the more obvious physical and sensory disabling conditions. Large numbers of children who do not exhibit any obvious physical or sensory abnormalities suffer various forms of mild disorders—behavioral, emotional, and intellectual—which affect their capacity to learn and perform age-appropriate skills. Concern for high drop-out rates in early primary grades in developing countries has increased in recent years (see Fobih, 1983 and Pollitt, 1980 for a discussion of this issue as it relates to Ghana and Latin America respectively). Although socioeconomic, cultural, and motivational factors may be the leading factors associated with school drop-out, it is highly conceivable that children with mild unnoticeable disorders account for quite a sizeable proportion of children who drop out of school in the early grades.

One of the propositions of this discussion is that mild forms of behavioral, emotional, and intellectual disorders among children may represent one manifestation of the residual effects of environmental factors related to high infant and early childhood mortality. That is, children who survive these early hazards may suffer long-term deleterious effects, however mild, on their ability to function and perform as normal children. Consequently, any attempt to understand the etiology of childhood disability in a developing country should include a critical examination of the most common causes of infant and early childhood mortality.

Epidemiological data from all over the developing world show overwhelmingly that the major causes of infant and early childhood mortality and morbidity are mainly preventable or curable pathogenic conditions which are concomitantly related to such qualities of poverty stricken environments as poor sanitation, poor drinking water, inadequate nutrition, poor housing, etc.

SPECIFIC CONDITIONS AND RELATED ETIOLOGICAL FACTORS

Most direct causes of childhood disability, like the more generalized causes of high mortality, derive from preventable conditions. Malnutrition, infections—viral, parasitic, or bacterial—and communicable as well as noncommunicable somatic diseases are responsible for well over 50% of disability cases. All over the world genetic disorders account for a very small proportion—less than 10%— of disabilities.

Inadequate nutrition is one of the most serious problems facing developing regions of the world today. Despite the largely agrarian economic base of most of these countries, misplaced priorities in development planning expose large numbers of infants/young children and their nursing mothers to varying degrees of undernutrition and malnutrition. A study published by the World Health Organization in 1978 which examined the social and biological correlates of perinatal mortality cited malnutrition as being responsible for up to 57% of infant deaths in some developing countries. Another major finding from epidemiological studies conducted in developing countries is the accentuation of the early childhood mortality rate due to the interaction between poor nutrition and infectious diseases. Examples of data on this interaction have been reported on Latin America (Morley, 1973; Puffer & Serrano, 1973) and Africa (Sanders, 1982).

The Latin American studies provide more insight into the extent to which malnutrition increases vulnerability to infections and accentuates case fatality rates. For example, Morley (1973) found that 62% of severely malnourished children, compared to 22% of normal children, experienced at least one episode of diarrhea each year. Morley reported also that undernourished children contracting measles showed a mortality rate 400 times higher than their well-nourished counterparts. The Puffer and Serrano (1973) survey reported similar findings; 57% of children under 5 who died exhibited signs of intrauterine and/or postnatal nutritional growth retardation as the primary or an associated cause of death.

The implications of the high incidence of malnutrition in developing countries are obvious; it has been known for many years that one of the most debilitating long-term effects of early childhood malnutrition is poor mental development. Investigations by Richardson and his associates in Jamaica (Richardson, Birch, & Hertzig, 1973; Richardson, Birch, & Ragbeer, 1975), Brockman and Riccuiti (1971) in Peru, Monckeberg (1968) in Chile, Cravioto and Robles (1965) in

Mexico, and by researchers at the Institute of Nutrition of Central America and Panama (INCAP) in Guatemala (Townsend, Klein, Irwin, Owens, Yarborough, & Engle, 1982) represent examples of efforts to study the impact of malnutrition on the mental development of children in the developing world. A longitudinal study of Jamaican children hospitalized for protein-energy malnutrition (PEM) found that about 6 to 8 years after their discharge from hospital these children manifested low IQ scores, lower school achievement, and more behavior problems than their normal peers of similar socioeconomic background. While several issues related to design and instrumentation render the interpretation of these findings a difficult exercise, the replication of findings across studies does suggest on the whole that poor mental development may result from the synergistic effects of nutrition deficiency and other conditions of extreme poverty.

In pregnant mothers, poor nutrition and starvation have marked deleterious effects on the developing foetus not only in terms of nutritional deprivation to the child but also in terms of increasing the mother's vulnerability to infections. Exposure of the foetus to infectious agents, such as malaria parasites and the rubella or measles viruses, is responsible for several types of nongenetic congenital malformations. Maternal malnutrition may also increase perinatal risks—e.g. difficult delivery due to maternal anaemia may result in damage to the child's central nervous system.

Among older infants and young children complications from several preventable infections due to poor health care may result in various disabling conditions. Infections of the central nervous system—e.g. cerebral malaria, spinal meningitis, and encephalitis—may lead to brain damage, hearing impairment, and cerebral palsy respectively. Viral infections like measles and mumps can also lead to damage to the brain and to impaired hearing. A recent study of 800 profoundly deaf children in 4 Nigerian states reported that while the probable cause of deafness could not be ascertained in one-third of the cases, almost all the remaining cases were caused by some preventable condition; measles accounted for 20% while meningitis accounted for 18% of cases (Holborow et al., 1981).

Poliomyelitis, another viral infection, is still one of the most crippling conditions in developing countries. In fact, contrary to what one might expect on the basis of current advancements in medical technology, this condition is on the increase in several developing countries. In Ghana (Addy & Otatumi, 1977; Korsah, 1983) and in the Indonesian province of Yogyakarta (Ulfah et al., 1981), polio has been reported as the most common cause of crippling in children. In the Indonesian study, the finding that 9 per 10,000 in the 0-20 year age group compared to 22 per 10,000 in the 1-3 year group led the authors to suggest that at least in that province there was an increasing trend in the incidence of paralytic polio. One report on the incidence of polio in Nigeria has indicated that the number of children with polio seen for treatment at the University of Ibadan Hospital rose from 3,142 in 1967 to 12,275 in 1975 (Commonwealth Foundation, 1977).

World Health Organization figures for 1978 showed a sharp increase in reported cases of polio in 22 African countries (Kenya for example reported more cases in 1978 than in any other previous year). Only 11 African countries observed a decrease in reported cases while two countries maintained zero incidence (in terms of reported cases). In WHO's Western Pacific region, Vietnam was reported in 1978 as having maintained an increasing trend in polio cases for five consecutive years. In a recent review of surveys done in Ghana, Egypt, Burma, and the Philippines, Sabin (1980) identifies paralytic polio as a serious threat in developing countries, and draws attention to the huge discrepancies between officially reported cases and survey-related prevalence rates. He cautions that in many developing countries, the prevalence of polio approaches, and in some cases far exceeds, the 100 per million total population rate found in the United States during the pre-vaccine era.

Two surveys of lameness among school children in Ghana reported data which yielded annual incidence rates of 280 per million (Nicholas et al., 1977) and 232 per million (Ofosu-Amaah et al., 1977) total population. In Burma, although the officially reported rate was 10 per million total population, a 1975 survey of primary school children in the Rangoon area reported data which yielded an incidence rate nearly six times the national estimate. In the Philippines, a 1976 survey revealed a "minimum annual average incidence of at least 145 paralytic poliomyelitis cases per million total population" (Sabin, 1980; p. 145). The data from all the above studies showed overwhelmingly that most of the children (about 95%) with paralytic polio suffered the condition during the first three years of life.

Blindness is a common disabling condition linked to several preventable environmental causes. An estimated 75% of the world's blind live in developing countries where trachoma, onchocerciasis (river blindness), and xerophthalmia (blindness from vitamin A deficiency), all preventable conditions, represent the major causes of visual impairments. It is estimated that in the Middle East alone, some 7.5 million people are blinded by trachoma and communicable eye diseases (WHO, 1979a), while in West Africa trachoma and onchocerciasis are the leading causes of blindness. In 1973 an estimated one million people in the Volta Basin of West Africa were reported to be affected by onchocerciasis. Although some progress towards prevention has been made since the Onchocerciasis Control Program was launched in 1975, total control of the black fly which transmits the disease has not been achieved after almost a decade of preventive activity. The role of nutritional deficiency in blindness is well illustrated by India where an estimated one quarter of a million children become blind each year through vitamin A deficiency. Zaman (Chapter 12 in this volume) reports that in Bangladesh 25,000 young children may be blinded each year through factors associated with nutritional deficiency.

As was pointed out earlier in the discussion, these preventable and/or curable environmental factors coupled with traumas and injuries—e.g. traffic, home, and other accidents—are responsible for well over 50% of the incidence of disability. The rationale for emphasising these variables in the preceding review of causes has been to demonstrate the potential amount of control that, given proper direction and planning, developing countries can have over childhood disability. In principle, if preventable causes are responsible for over 50% of incidence, then effective preventive measures should lead to a reduction of the incidence of disability by at least one-half. Additionally, a sizeable proportion of childhood disability could be avoided if effective health and medical services are in place to provide secondary prevention in the form of drug treatment of disabling diseases or corrective surgery for congenital orthopaedic conditions.

APPRAISAL OF EXISTING HEALTH CARE SYSTEMS

Prevention versus cure: It is obvious from the foregoing analysis that any comprehensive health care delivery system in developing countries should have a strong preventive component. A major conclusion which often emerges from health and epidemiological surveys in developing countries is that these countries require a health care system which will effectively prevent suffering, disability, or death from easily preventable diseases among infants and young children. Despite this realization, the western model of health care with its heavy emphasis on curative medicine remains the dominant approach to health care delivery in most developing countries. Aidoo (1982) cites data on Ghana which illustrate the near absence of emphasis on preventive medicine. In 1970 only 3.5% of the 565 doctors practising in Ghana were in preventive medicine. Aidoo further cites evidence from Ghana's Five-Year Development Plan indicating that in the 1973-74 financial year only 13.3% of the total expenditure on health went into preventive medicine compared to 77.1% for curative medical care. During the three-year period 1973/74 to 1975/76, the budgetary allocation for preventive medicine diminished by 3.6 percentage points compared to a 1.2 percentage-point reduction in the allocation for curative medical services.

Much of the preventive work taking place in developing countries today represents initiatives by international organizations. All the massive immunization programs (e.g. the Smallpox Eradication Program involving some 20 West and Central African countries in the late 60s and early 70s) and vector control projects (e.g. prevention of river blindness in the Volta Basin of West Africa) have been implemented through external initiatives. A World Health Organization report (WHO, 1979b) emphasizing the need for increased commitment to the eradication of common fatal childhood diseases noted that only 10% of the 80 million children born annually in developing countries receive immunization. Consequently, 5 million children die each year while another 5 million are crippled, mentally retarded or otherwise disabled for life by such preventable diseases as diphtheria, pertusis (whooping cough), tetanus, measles, polio, and tuberculosis. The report noted further that despite these alarming statistics, "in the developing countries the diseases are so commonplace that parents, health workers, and political leaders have come to accept the continuing existence of this tragic situation" (WHO, 1979b; p. 128) as a normal way of life.

Although the World Health Organization, through its Expanded Program on Immunization (EPI), hopes to achieve the immunization of every child against those six childhood diseases by 1990, the program's long term objective of making immunization services a permanent component of primary health care cannot be achieved without commitment from indigenous governments of the developing world. It is not being suggested that indigenous governments have not shown commitment to programs of this nature at all. However, whatever commitment has been shown has not been sufficiently reflected in the long-term planning of health needs and goals in individual nations.

Rural-urban discrepancies: Although the population of most developing countries is largely rural in character, with as much as 70 to 80 per cent of the adult population and even a higher proportion of children living in rural and peri-urban communities, the characteristically urban-oriented national development policies of individual nations have resulted in a disproportionate concentration of services and infrastructure in large urban centres. Perhaps no area better demonstrates the irrationality that characterizes development planning in some developing countries than the provision of health and sanitation services.

That the quality of life is lower among the rural majority is a fact borne out by social and epidemiological research and often acknowledged in preambles to national development planning policy statements. The differences in the quality of life between urban and rural communities are overwhelmingly replicated in research throughout the developing world. One survey done in pre-independence Zimbabwe in 1976 (see Sanders, 1982) reported variations in infant mortality rates from as low as 21 per 1,000 in the capital city to as high as 300 per 1,000 live births in a remote western district. During the same period an OXFAM report indicated that as much as 80% of children in rural areas were undernourished (Sanders, 1982). This survey is of utmost socio-political importance in its illustration of the colonial roots of the predominantly urban-oriented political economies of many developing countries.

In Ghana a 1978 survey of health needs and health services carried out by the Institute of Development Studies in Brighton (Aidoo, 1982) and a Ministry of Health report released in the same year revealed similar rural-urban discrepancy patterns in indices of the quality of life. While the infant mortality rate for the national capital was 63 per 1,000 live births, the average for rural areas was over 100 per 1,000. In fact, a rate as high as 234 per 1,000 has been reported in the Upper Region (one of the remotest areas) of the country (Ghana Ministry of Health, 1978).

Based upon the kind of data reviewed here—which are replicated in most developing countries and are readily available to governments—one would expect rural populations to be given greater attention in health care planning and delivery than is currently available. This, however, is not the case in most developing countries. Using Ghana, again, to illustrate this point, between 1970 and 1976 40% of the country's health budget was spent on tertiary health care, mainly in the large regional and other urban hospitals serving no more than 10% of the population (Ghana Ministry of Health, 1978). Primary health care needed by some 90% of the population attracted only 15% of budgetary expenditures. In fact, in the 1973/74 financial year, expenditure on the Korle Bu Teaching Hospital alone (the nation's largest hospital located in the capital) represented 12% of the total health budget (Aidoo, 1982). In terms of health personnel allocation in Ghana, Twumasi (1975) reports that only 24% of health personnel and 14% of doctors registered with the Ministry of Health were stationed in rural areas. Data on the Indian state of Maharashtra during the same period showed that 80% of that state's health care expenditures was spent on three cities, although the vast majority of the population lived in rural areas (Mangudkar, 1978). In terms of sanitation services, WHO data collected from all over the world during the 1970-75 period showed that 78% of the population in rural areas lacked an adequate supply of water while 85% lacked satisfactory sanitation services (WHO, 1979b).

This concentration of social amenities and services in urban centres is partially responsible for the rural-urban drift so characteristic of developing countries. Rural dwellers are leaving the countryside in their large numbers to seek better economic opportunities and a better future which they hope to find in the cities. Such modern amenities and social services as better health care and educational facilities, better drinking water, electricity, and so on, make the cities more attractive than the largely neglected rural areas. Ironically, however, these "attractions" are not only becoming "extinct species" in many cities in the developing world but where they exist at all they are not easily available to the new migrant peri-urban dwellers who continue to live in abject conditions of poverty. The implications of the rural-urban migration process, sometimes reaching exodus proportions, include the collapse of the rural agricultural sector, the proliferation of import-oriented urban commercial activity, and the resultant food shortages which, in turn, often give rise to malnutrition, disease, and disability.

THE FALLACY OF 'UNIDIRECTIONAL CAUSAL RELATIONSHIPS'

The relationship between indices of socio-economic status on one hand and mortality and morbidity rates on the other is well established in the social science and epidemiological literature. To cite a few studies conducted in the developing world, Carvajal and Burgess (1978) analyzed data from an urban fertility survey sponsored in the

1960s by the UN Centre for Latin American Demography in order to test the hypothesis that the occurrence of fetal and child deaths in three Latin American cities—Bogota (Colombia), Caracas (Venezuela), and Rio de Janeiro (Brazil)—was sytematically influenced by parental socio-economic environment. The researchers found that fetal mortality was more prevalent in lower income groups than it was in higher income groups. This major finding was explained by a number of related findings; for example, malnutrition and lack of sanitation services were found to occur more often in lower than in higher income families.

In a study of malnutrition among children in a rural area of Bangladesh, Bairagi (1980) reported that while the important determinants of malnutrition included seasonal factors (e.g. during the harvest season 15% of children were severely malnourished compared to 26% during the lean season), family income and mother's education were both significantly related to children's nutritional status for both the lean and the bumper seasons. These findings present several dimensions of the problem of malnutrition. The seasonal differences in the incidence of severe malnutrition suggests that availability of food is an important factor in malnutrition. However, the socio-economic variations reported suggest also that unequal access to food, and possibly, differences in socio-cultural nutritional practices and values may be additional critical factors.

More recently Cochrane and Mehra (1983) have reported data on Africa which confirm a strong inverse relationship between child mortality and the socio-economic variable maternal education. Their data on ten countries—Ethiopia, Gambia, Ghana, Kenya, Senegal, Sierra Leone, Sudan, Tanzania, Uganda, and Zambia—show unequivocally that during infancy and early childhood (birth to 5 years) the mortality rate is highest among infants and young children whose mothers have the least education. Cochrane and Mehra have concluded:

> *Even a small amount of education (one to three years) is significant in reducing child mortality...In many countries, the most educated women have a mortality rate of their children that is less than half the rate of the least educated women (p. 28).*

For example in Ethiopia 18% of children in the birth to 2-year group whose mothers had no school education at all died compared to 13.7% and 1.2% for children of the same age whose mothers had elementary and above elementary education respectively. In Gambia, Ghana, Sierra Leone, and Uganda where the child mortality rates were generally higher, children of mothers with more than elementary school education showed a mortality rate some 15 percentage points lower than the rate for children of mothers who had no formal education.

Education is perhaps the most frequently examined socio-economic index because it appears to be an easier-to-obtain measure compared to other socioeconomic variables. It is important to stress, however, that in the developing countries especially, education is also highly related to such other socio-economic variables as income, urban residence, and improved knowledge of and access to medical facilities. Thus there is a demonstrated relationship between socio-economic variables and indices of the quality of life. The question arises, however, as to whether this relationship is merely correlational or causal as well.

From an empirical-statistical point of view, the reported data including Cochrane and Mehra's results are correlational in nature and do not permit any causal inferences to be made. However, the dominant model of national development planning in many developing countries is one that appears to assume that many of the social problems related to poverty could be eliminated simply by increasing economic productivity. This notion of development as a primarily economic process implies a unidirectional causal relationship between economic productivity and social well-being. The consequence of this notion has been an increasing tendency to ignore persistent challenges to institute social welfare programs under the pretext of building a strong economic base that will ultimately lead to improved quality of life.

While recognizing the crucial role of increased productivity in both economic and social progress, this chapter takes the view that the unidirectional causal relationship assumption inherent in development planning strategies which emphasize economic productivity in the hope of automatically producing a panacea for social problems related to poverty is at best parochial. In fact contemporary experiences from oil producing countries in the developing world as well as the Latin American experience of the early 1970s show clearly that significant economic development per se does not necessarily reduce poverty and human misery for the majority of the people. A political philosophy founded upon equity, social justice, and the reduction of human misery is a crucial prerequisite if economic development is to culminate in comprehensive national programs that will ultimately alleviate poverty and human suffering for the majority of the people.

From a conceptual-theoretical perspective any valid hypothesis of causal relationship between economic productivity and social well-being must be bidirectional. In the context of the present discussion, the bidirectional causal relationship between poverty, disease and disability on one hand and economic productivity on the other is exemplified in Gaston de Merzerville's (1979) model which describes the circular relationship between underdevelopment and social problems. The model illustrates very well the point that a strategy of national development planning which relegates the development of human services to a low priority status can be potentially counterproductive. Underdevelopment, according to the model, is characterized by low economic productivity and leads to poor diets, malnutrition, and disease. Disease, in turn, may produce higher morbidity, disability, and lower life expectancy, all of which are factors causally related to low productivity and underdevelopment. In investment terms, high incidence of disease forces a nation, in the face of limited resources, to invest more in curative medical care at the expense of preventive and promotional programs, a situation which produces a vicious cycle of more illness and impairment, higher disability rates, low productivity, and underdevelopment.

The costs to the developing world of a large population of disabled children are enormous. In economic terms, the erosion of human capital resulting from disability and allied problems constitutes a phenomenal impediment to socioeconomic development. In educational terms, the prevalence of mild forms of developmental disabilities manifesting themselves in behavioral, emotional, and mild intellectual disorders in school-age children does not place such children well to fully gain the potential benefits of education. The boomerang effect of this situation, in economic terms, is to minimize the return to society of investments on education (Austin, 1976).

THE SOLUTION: TREATMENT OR REFORM?

The rationale for focusing on the preventable ecological causes of disease and disability, while pursuing an analysis of the bidirectional causal relationship between economic productivity and social well-being, is to emphasize the need for developing countries to look beyond the medical model of disease for a better understanding of the problem of childhood disability. The economic, political, and socio-cultural ecologies should be seen as major etiological variables as well as crucial keys to successful intervention. The health care scenario described in the preceding sections shows that rural dwellers upon whom poverty makes its most devastating impact are also the least protected in terms of their health and other social welfare needs. Considering that rural dwellers constitute the vast majority of the population in most developing countries and produce the bulk of the national wealth, this situation represents a critical socio-political problem. It is the contention of this author that increasing disease and disability rates are concomitantly endemic to political economies which are not founded upon social justice, equity, and broad-based development planning. Consequently, a change in socio-political orientation is a *sine qua non* if morbidity and mortality rates are to be reduced and the quality of life improved for the majority of the developing world's population.

The solution to the health care and social welfare problems of the developing world should no longer be seen in a *treatment approach* (the provision of token services for temporary relief from symptoms of bigger underlying problems) but in a *reform approach* which seeks to correct broader structural political and socioeconomic defects and/or imbalances. Strategies of national development need to be broadbased and to reflect the realization of the imperative to make a direct attack on poverty and its social manifestations—malnutrition, disease, disability, poor shelter, poor environmental sanitation, etc.

An ecological approach is proposed as the most rational and practical way to attain not only the specific goals of preventing childhood disability but also to achieve the broader goals towards overall improvement of the quality of life. The ecological approach is the process whereby economic and social-political actions are integrated to create within the natural and social-cultural ecologies conditions which will promote optimum quality of life. The approach is founded on a premise emphasized in an earlier paper (Marfo, 1983) and reiterated in the present discussion, namely that the high incidence of disease and disability among children in the developing world is related, at least in part, to the inheritance and perpetuation of dysfunctional political and economic systems which inherently create and maintain wide social and economic disparities between the advantaged minority and the disadvantaged majority. Thus the solution to the problem of childhood disability, which is also a solution to general health problems, depends as much on the ability of governments in the developing world to carry out structural political and economic reforms as it does on its ability to implement specific community-based intervention programs.

However, it is important to point out, as Sidel and Sidel (1977) have rightly observed with specific reference to primary health care, that the quest for improved quality of life—through effective and cost-efficient methods founded on the principles of equity and social justice—can itself constitute a leading edge for change in the socio-political structure. In fact, the strength of an ecological approach to disability prevention lies in its long-term potential to bring this change about by emphasizing the interrelationships that exist among society's natural (physical), social-cultural, economic, and political ecologies.

Central to an ecological approach are two related views about health: (a) good quality health cannot be attained through the traditionally known formal health sector alone; and (b) health care means more than curative medicine (Buri, 1982). First, good health is a function of a total environment which is free of health problems, and the attainment of this kind of environment depends on the integrated efforts of several sectors of national planning—agriculture, social welfare, public works, education, information, and health. Second, health care itself embraces curative as well as preventive, promotive, rehabilitative, and community development activities.

With particular reference to the prevention of disability in early childhood, the need for increased emphasis upon preventive medicine becomes imperative. Such preventive medical action should, however, be integrated with social action to ensure total eradication of the myriad environmental conditions which necessitate preventive medical action in the first place. Integrated community development and community-based social action programming utilizing local human and material resources are, consequently, important dimensions of an ecological approach. On a more philosophical level, development planning activities and specific social action programs should be guided by the courage to be indigenous in adopting strategies best suited for dealing with the problems of the developing world. The major goals of integrated community development activities should therefore include:

- providing adequate and good quality water supply;
- improving sanitation services;
- striving towards self sufficiency in the production of a wide variety of indigenous food items necessary to ensure balanced nutrition;
- improving inter-village communication links through road construction, and as a means of increasing accessibility to major food

producing areas, etc.

These are primary human needs and services without which many of the more formal health programs are likely to fail. These formal health programs include the provision of rural health posts/centres, the development and implementation of comprehensive immunization programs, the training of village health workers, the training and/or reorientation of traditional birth attendants within broader maternal and child health (MCH) programs, and health and nutrition education.

In effect, an ecological approach is consistent with and acknowledges primary health care—as proposed and defined by the World Health Organization—as a potential panacea not only for the growing threat of childhood disability in particular, but also for the general health problems which confront the developing world.

Having acknowledged the principle of primary health care, it should be pointed out that primary health care has unfortunately been assigned a rather superficial meaning not only by governments to whom the notion has been recommended but even sometimes by the recommending and advising experts. The original conceptualization of primary health care views the approach in a very broad *ecological* perspective. For example, the World Health Organization has emphasized that "the most important single factor in promoting primary health care and overcoming obstacles is a strong political will and support at both national and community levels, reinforced by a firm national strategy." (WHO, 1979c; p. 448). Regarding the need for an inter-sectoral approach to health care planning, WHO further notes:

> *In developing countries in particular, economic development anti-poverty measures, food production, water, sanitation, housing, environmental protection and education all contribute to health and have the same goal of human development. Primary health care, as an integral part of the health system and of overall social and economic development, will of necessity rest on proper coordination at all levels between the health and other sectors concerned. (p. 448).*

However, despite the laudable efforts of the World Health Organization, in very few countries can concrete evidence be found of systematic and long-term efforts to make primary health care an integral part of national development strategies. In many other places PHC has not gone beyond a few isolated demonstration or pilot projects—

largely in the traditional health sector—in selected communities. While such experimental projects continue to yield excellent data on the extent to which PHC can improve the quality of life, the implementation of the scheme on a national scale backed by long-term planning, as well as the coordination between health and other sectors of development, remain a distant objective.

The future emphases are clear. As long as poverty, malnutrition, and preventable infectious diseases continue to plague the developing world no hope exists for curbing the rising trends in the incidence of childhood disability. And as the population of our disabled children continually increases, the burden to habilitate and rehabilitate will become even bigger, and the proportion of disabled persons receiving rehabilitation services—already very small—will become even smaller as a function of our limited resources. The onus lies on professionals within the developing world as well as on international organizations to emphasize the need to make a direct attack on the environmental causes of disability. A dollar spent on prevention may be worth several hundreds saved in future habilitation and rehabilitation expenses.

It is heartening to note that over the past five years or so, remarkable strides have been made on the international scene in the promotion of disability prevention and early intervention programs. International organizations principally involved in these efforts include the WHO, UNICEF, UNDP, and Rehabilitation International (RI). In 1981 RI, in its *Charter for the 80s*, committed itself to launching "in each nation a program to prevent as many impairments as possible and to ensure that the necessary preventive services reach every family and every person." Since then RI has been working actively with UNICEF and other agencies in the area of disability prevention.

UNICEF, WHO, and UNDP have increased their commitment to disability prevention in recent years by jointly launching and supporting IMPACT, the United Nations interagency program for disability prevention. In several parts of the developing world today, these organizations are working actively with indigenous governments in implementing preventive, early intervention, and/or community rehabilitation programs. Hammerman (1984) attributes recent country level expansions in disability prevention programs to several factors, including the fact that the kind of interagency collaboration referred to above has become more intense and focused over the past few years. An additional factor appears to be related to the impact on individual national governments of numerous international activities associated with the International Year of Disabled Persons (1981) and the Decade of Disabled Persons (1983-1992).

The following brief overview of program activities, based on reports by Hammerman (1984) and Rao and O'Dell (1984), should serve to inform the reader about recent advances at the international scene.

In Asia and the Pacific region, where perhaps the majority of UNICEF assisted community based prevention and rehabilitation programs are in place, program objectives include the following:

- to assess, through basic data collection, the extent and magnitude of the problem of childhood disability and of the situation of disabled children;
- to increase family and community awareness of the problems and needs of disabled children;
- to provide support and assistance to nongovernmental organizations (NGOs) currently engaged in innovative, cost-effective, and replicable programs;
- to assist in the training of teachers, community workers, and parents in prevention, early detection and management;
- to promote and/or engage in research and development activity, in collaboration with governments and NGOs, aimed at identifying effective strategies for prevention, early detection, and community based rehabilitation.

In India, some of UNICEF's achievements include assistance to the Ministry of Social Welfare and some 30 NGOs in various activities, including the integration of community based actions into the Indian Integrated Child Development program which covers more than 100 million people (Hammerman, 1984). Recently, UNICEF commissioned a 5-part childhood disability film for parents and professionals and produced a sound-slide on polio immunization (Rao & O'Dell, 1984).

In Sri Lanka, a district development project is underway in which an integrated program for disability prevention and community based rehabilitation is being implemented, and in Nepal a similar project has already produced an information kit (the Nepal Kit) for community rehabilitation workers based on the RI/UNICEF manual.

In the Philippines, UNICEF has been assisting in the local adaptation and field testing of the WHO Community Rehabilitation training manual (Hammerman, 1984). As Miles (Chapter 7 in this volume) reports, in Pakistan the Community Rehabilitation scheme has been field tested in the Punjab while in the North West Frontier, a FAMH/UNICEF Community Rehabilitaion Development project has been implemented with support from the government.

In the Africa region where childhood disability prevention activity is fairly recent, phenomenal progress has been made in a relatively short period. In November 1984, program IMPACT was officially launched in Nairobi, Kenya. Prior to this event, however, data gathering to assess the magnitude of childhood disability had been initiated in Botswana, Zambia, and Zimbabwe. Some of the results of the Zambia survey have already been published in the African Rehabilitation Journal (see Davies, 1983) and the International Rehabilitation Review. One of the positive outcomes of the Zambia study was UNICEF's decision in 1984 "to intensify the medical outreach services and the community based rehabilitation efforts" (Hammerman, 1984; p. 9) to those children identified in the survey.

In Botswana, an innovative program is currently being supported by UNICEF and the Van Leer Foundation to put in place a country-wide training program for mothers which will teach child survival and child development concepts. Already there is a UNICEF-sponsored project on the detection of childhood disability which includes workshops for primary school teachers. In Ethiopia, both UNICEF and the ILO are assisting in the training of Community Rehabilitation Aides (CRAs).

In other parts of the developing world, programs with similar emphases are being implemented with the support of UNICEF and other international organizations. In Chapter 4 Thorburn covers several programs in the Caribbean that are currently supported by UNICEF and other international organizations. The stability and ultimate success of these programs will depend upon the extent to which indigenous governments and NGOs embrace and incorporate them into their long term development plans. It is hoped that these international organizations will continue to emphasize the need for local actions to sustain and expand these programs.

CONCLUSION

In the foregoing discussion the relationship between increasing disability rates and poor or inadequate health care planning and delivery in the developing countries has been stressed. More importantly, however, both the increasing trends in the incidence of disability and inadequate health care services have been portrayed as representing a concomitant manifestation of strategies of national development planning which fail to respond to the needs of the majority of the developing world's surging population. This characterization of the problem necessarily places emphasis on the relationship between political systems and socio-economic planning on one hand, and social well-being or quality of life on the other. The past decade has witnessed a phenomenal growth of awareness of this relationship and of the crucial need to deal with it. The leadership of the World Health Organization in the promotion of primary health care, especially since the Alma Ata declaration of 1978, is a practical demonstration of efforts to confront the developing world's health problems. Since 1981, the World Bank, for instance, has been expanding its lending program for health to assist and strengthen primary health care systems. The Bank sees its policy expansion in this direction as an essential step if the problems of poverty and low productivity among the poor are to be dealt with effectively (World Bank, 1980). The Bank's emphasis on *preventive medicine* is particularly noteworthy.

Just as curative medicine has received more attention than preventive medicine and health promotion, habilitation and rehabilitation of the disabled continue to take precedence over disability prevention. However, the prevention imperative is far too obvious to ignore. The major steps to confronting childhood disability in developing countries should be seen as falling on a directional continuum beginning with primary prevention. In this connection, immunization and vector control programs as well as health promotion through environmental sanitation and other community development activities should feature strongly in long-term national development strategies. The leadership currently provided by UNICEF, WHO, UNDP, RI, and other international organizations in the area of prevention and community rehabilitation should serve to challenge governments and agencies in developing countries to make disability prevention a major priority in coming decades.

References

Aidoo, T.A. (1982). Rural health under colonialism and neocolonialism: A survey of the Ghanaian experience. *International Journal of Health Service,* **12**, 637-657.

Addy, P.A.K. & Otatumi, S. (1977). Poliovirus serotypes 1 and 2: The major cause of infantile paralysis in Ghana—1972 through 1974. *Ghana Medical Journal,* **16**, 61-62.

Austin, J. E. (1976). *Urban malnutrition: Problems, assessment, and intervention guides.* Cambridge, Mass.: Harvard University Press.

Bairagi, R. (1980). Is income the only constraint on child nutrition in rural Bangladesh? *Bulletin of the World Health Organization, 58,* 767-772.

Brockman, L., & Riccuiti, H. (1971). Severe protein-calorie malnutrition and cognitive development in infancy and early childhood. *Developmental Psychology, 4*, 312-316.

Buri, R. (1982). Health care or medical care—Guest editorial. *Public Health Reviews, X*(3-4), 223-227.

Carvajal, M. & Burgess, P. (1978). Socioeconomic status and child deaths in Latin America: A comparative study of Bogota, Caracas, and Rio de Janeiro. *Social Science and Medicine, 12c*, 89-98.

Cochrane, S. & Mehra, K. (1983). Socioeconomic determinants of infant and child mortality in developing countries. *Child Development and International Development,* **No. 20**, 27-43.

Commonwealth Foundation. (1977). *The disabled in developing countries: A symposium.* London: Commonwealth Foundation.

Cravioto, J., & Robles, B. (1965). Evolution of adaptive and motor behavior during rehabilitation from Kwashiokor. *American Journal of Orthopsychiatry, 35*, 449-452.

Davies, M. (1983). The Zimbabwe national disability survey. *The African Rehabilitation Journal, 1*(1), 18-21.

Djukanovic, V. & Mach, E.P. (Eds.), (1975). *Alternative approaches to meeting basic health needs in developing countries.* Geneva: World Health Organization.

Fobih, D.K. (1983). A model for a preschool programme and its relevance to the education of the disabled in Ghana. In K. Marfo, S. Walker, & B.L. Charles (Eds.), *Education and rehabilitation of the disabled in Africa, Vol. 1: Towards improved services.* Edmonton: University of Alberta Centre for International Education and Development.

Ghana Ministry of Health. (1978). *A primary health care strategy for Ghana.* Accra: Ministry of Health Planning Unit.

Gwatkins, D.R. (1979). *The end of an era: Recent evidence indicates an unexpected early showing of mortality in many developing countries.* Washington, D.C.: Overseas Development Council.

Hammerman, S. (1984). UNICEF involvement in disability prevention, early intervention programs. *International Rehabilitation Review, 3rd & 4th Quarter,* 9.

Holborow, C., Martinson, F., & Anger, N. (1981). A study of deafness in West Africa. *Commonwealth Society for the Deaf Occasional Paper.*

Korsah, K.G. (1983). Integration of health services for the rehabilitation of the disabled in Ghana. In K. Marfo, S. Walker, & B.L. Walker (Eds.), *Education and rehabilitation of the disabled in Africa, Vol. 1: Towards improved services.* Edmonton: University of Alberta Centre for International Education and Development.

Mangudkar, M. P. (1978). *Health for the millions (Vol. IV, No. 5)* New Delhi: Voluntary Health Association.

Marfo, K. (1983). Community-based approaches to disability prevention and early habilitation in the context of developing countries. *University of Alberta Centre for International Education and Development Occasional Paper Series, No. 2.*

de Merzerville, G. (1979). *Disability and rehabilitation in rural Costa Rica.* East Lansing, Michigan: University Centres for International Rehabilitation.

Monckeberg, F. (1968). Effect of early marasmic malnutrition on subsequent physical and psychological development. In N. S. Scrimshaw & L. Gordon (Eds.), *Malnutrition, learning and behavior.* Cambridge, Mass.: MIT Press.

Morley, D. (1973). *Pediatric priorities in the developing world.* London: Butterworths.

Nicholas, D. D., Kratzer, J. H., Ofosu-Amaah, S., & Belcher, D. W. (1977). Is poliomyelitis a serious problem in developing countries?—The Danfa experience. *British Medical Journal, 1,* 1009-1012.

Noble, J.H. (1981). Social inequity in the prevalence of disability—Projections for the year 2000. *Assignment Children,* **53/54**, 23-32.

Ofosu-Amaah, S., Kratzer, J. H., & Nicholas, D. D. (1977). Is poliomyelitis a serious problem in developing countries?—Lameness in Ghanaian schools. *British Medical Journal, 1,* 1012-1014.

Pollitt, E. (1980). *Poverty and malnutrition in Latin America: Early childhood intervention programs.* New York: Praeger Publishers.

Puffer, R. R., & Serrano, C. V. (1973). *Patterns of child mortality in childhood.* Washington, D.C.: Pan American Health Organization (Scientific Publication No. 262).

Rao, A., & O'Dell, D. (1984, June). *The UNICEF experience in India.* Paper presented at the 15th World Congress of Rehabilitation International, Lisbon, Portugal.

Richardson, S.A., Birch, H.G., & Hertzig, M.E. (1973). School performance of children who were severely malnourished in infancy. *American Journal of Mental Deficiency,* **77**, 623.

Richardson, S.A., Birch, H., & Ragbeer, C. (1975). The behavior of children at home who were severely malnourished in the first two years of life. *Journal of Biosocial Science,* 7, 255.

Sabin, A. B. (1980). Vaccination against poliomyelitis in economically underdeveloped countries. *Bulletin of the World Health Organization, 58*, 141-157.

Sanders, D. (1982). Nutrition and the use of food as a weapon in Zimbabwe and Southern Africa. *International Journal of Health Services,* **12**, 201-213.

Sidel, V. W., & Sidel, R. (1977). Primary health care in relation to socio-political structure. *Social Science and Medicine, 11*, 415-419.

Townsend, J.W., Klein, R.E., Irwin, M.H., Owens, W., Yarborough, C., & Engle, P. (1982). Nutrition and preschool mental development. In D.A. Wagner & H.W. Stevenson (Eds.), *Cultural perspectives on child development.* San Francisco: W.H. Freeman Company.

Twumasi, P.A. (1975). *Medical systems in Ghana: A study in medical sociology.* Tema: Ghana Publishing Corporation.

Ulfah, N. M., Parastho, S., Sadjimin, T., & Rhode, J. E. (1981). Polio and lameness in Yogyakarta, Indonesia. *International Journal of Epidemiology, 10*, 171-175.

WHO (1979a). Data on blindness throughout the world. *WHO Chronicle, 33*, 275-283.

WHO (1979b). Saving lives by immunization. *WHO Chronicle, 33*, 128-130.

WHO (1979c)Science and technology for health promotion in developing countries: 2. *WHO Chronicle, 33*, 447-556.

WHO (1980). *Sixth report on the world health situation—Part One: Global analysis.* Geneva: World Health Organization.

Wood, P.H.N. & Bradley, E.M. (1980). *People with disabilities.* New York: World Rehabilitation Fund.

World Bank (1980). *Health sector report, 2nd ed.* Washington, D.C.: World Bank Publications.

2

SCREENING FOR DEVELOPMENTAL DISABILITIES IN DEVELOPING COUNTRIES: PROBLEMS AND PERSPECTIVES

Tom Fryers[1]

Issues relating to disability in developing countries, have received scant attention until recently. Prevention of childhood illness and mortality has been given proper emphasis, but these problems are not truly separable from their disabling sequellae amongst survivors. The International Year of the Disabled Persons (IYDP) in 1981 seemed to focus attention at last on this situation and has resulted in widespread debate and some major publications (e.g Hammerman & Maikowski, 1981).

Studies of childhood disability in developing communities pose many difficulties, especially if they are to be useable beyond the community of origin. The results of work in highly developed countries is inevitably of questionable relevance. Do similar phenomena exist in different communities? Are they conceived and percieved in similar ways? Are they recognized as posing 'problems' of similar significance to the community? Do culturally normative interpretations of 'cause', both how and why, impose peculiar local constraints on action? Can they be measured in standardized ways, and is it worth making the attempt? Even in developed countries the field has been relatively little cultivated, and only very recently has a satisfactory terminology for 'impairment', 'disability', and 'handicap' been agreed upon and promulgated (WHO, 1980).

Current health priorities for developing countries are likely to remain for some time: guaranteeing adequate standards of nutrition for the whole population, largely through improvements in local agriculture; control of communicable diseases through public health

---

[1]This chapter is partly based upon 'Problems in screening for mental retardation in developing countries', published in the International Journal of Mental Health, 1981, 10(1).

measures; and the equitable distribution of health care resources through an appropriate primary health care infrastructure. There can also be little doubt that the most effective determinant of improved health of communities is generalized economic and social development. All these are relevant to the prevention of impairment and the limitation of disability and handicap, but thought needs to be given as to how to maximize benefits most efficiently for people who in most communities tend to be forgotten, ignored, or despised.

In particular, primary health care and primary education need to incorporate specific goals and tasks for disabled children and adults, to minimize handicap and maximize opportunites to participate in community life and enjoy the opportunities and choices afforded to their more able brothers and sisters. One contribution to this is through specific screening programs to detect disabling diseases, identify disabled children, and prescribe simple habilitation and rehabilitation programs which can be achieved within the community—e.g. those illustrated in the World Health Organization manual, *Training the disabled in the community* (Helander, Mendis, & Nelson, 1980).

We must beware of implying that all 'developing countries' are in some way the same: they probably differ far more than highly developed countries in demography, environment, history, and culture. We may expect them to share many consequences of a relative lack of resources, and low priority to the problems of disability but to vary considerably in the consequences of the processes of 'development' itself. Although some causes of serious impairment can be expected to diminish with improved health care and economic conditions, in many societies the high toll of infant mortality will particularly affect the most vulnerable children. As infant mortality decreases, so overtly impaired children are likely to survive in greater numbers and become much more prominent. However, the need to acknowledge the special problems of disabled children will naturally increase as the extension of primary education, industrialization, and urbanisation of society increase the demands upon, and the expectations of all children. Apart from any other local characteristics therefore, the prevalence of disabilites, especially those of early origin, will tend to vary with developmental status. The appropriateness of screening for any particular disorder, or serious impairments in general, will thus similarly vary.

SCREENING, MONITORING AND DIAGNOSIS

The term 'screening' has often been used exclusively for the application of simple tests to unselected or known high risk populations to identify positive indicators or pre-conditions of disease or disorder, but there is no fundamental distinction from many aspects of good clinical practice. Health workers, especially in primary health care settings, routinely examine babies, monitor pregnant women, and check contacts for infectious diseases. In all clinical contacts the conscientious worker will be alert to possibilities beyond the immediate subject of consultation. A two stage screening program, with a simple maneuver applied broadly to select a high risk group for detailed examination, is likely to be too expensive for most developing communities, and resources for detailed diagnosis are unlikely to be widely available. This emphasizes the importance of a satisfactory primary health care context.

Research in the pursuit of knowledge alone is hard to justify in poor communities, but screening may serve several pragmatic purposes. First is to offer practical help to those identified as disabled, principally by identitying and mobilizing community resources (Ng'andu & Sinyangwe, 1981). Second is to identify specific causes of disability susceptible to preventive action in that community for future generations (Paul, 1981). Third is to make visible the size and character of the problem to governments, administrators, professionals, community leaders and the people (Stein, 1981). Fourth is to provide statistical information for those who plan services and provide resources.

As has already been said, major differences exist between communities in different countries, cultures and environments. In the context of health care as much as anything, we have learnt, often too late, that giving too much weight to the wisdom of 'the West' and generalizing from their experience is frequently inappropriate, wasteful and dangerous. There are necessarily fundamental conceptual and practical difficulties in attempting to design screening instruments or to plan procedures for general application. Culture as well as linguistic translation will be a minimum requirement for success. Since the spectrum of disorders will vary so much from place to place, screening needs will also vary, and too rigid standardization may seriously prejudice relevance. Nevertheless, there are standard criteria for evaluating screening techniques and programs which should provide a satisfactory framework for discusssing the issues involved. They are conveniently expressed in question form.

CRITERIA FOR EFFECTIVE SCREENING

1. Is the disorder important? For the individual and family the presence of serious disability cannot be questioned, but the social and economic burden on particular communities will be largely determined by the local prevalence of each disability. This depends upon both incidence and survival. Where there is evidence of significant numbers of severely disabled children, it is important to identify them for treatment, care and rehabilitation as appropriate, and screening programs may easily be justified by early case finding. It is also necessary to establish fairly accurately the extent and nature of the community health problem to enable plans to be formulated for preventive, therapeutic and rehabilitative intervention on a community scale. For example, poliomyelitis is common in many African communities and it is possible to generalize on the need and preventive effectiveness of immunization, but because overtly disabled children do not get into schools and are effectively hidden in the community, comprehensive screening may be the only way of making contact with those already paralyzed, raising community awareness of their needs and potential, and establishing a practical program of community-based rehabilitation which exploits community resources in their interests, and prevents further disability and handicap. There will be many communities for which the same is true as regards severely retarded children, but many others where very few such vulnerable children survive early infancy, and the problem remains largely for the future, always remembering that rapidly changing societies may achieve that future quite soon.

2. Is there available a test, procedure or examination with which to recognize the target disorder? This is not as simple a question as may first appear; defining the target condition is fraught with difficulty and must be approached differently for different types of disability. This equally applies to the design or selection of screening procedures, especially where relatively untrained personnel are administering tests in village communities. For example, in the Zambia National Campaign to Reach Disabled Children it was found that hearing and seeing could be tested by simplified standard performance tests but orthopaedic disorders required structured observations of mobility, for example, and mental retardation required a structured interview with a parent or sibling (Parekh & Serpell, 1983). In order to devise a test that could be applied widely in many different populations we have to be clear about what we are really testing for. The problems are readily illustrated by reference to severe mental retardation (Fryers, 1984). Screening should give clear positive and negative results but unfortunately, it is not a unitary disorder but a pragmatic classification of variable definition and application. With intervention in mind for positive cases, target disorders can be defined in several ways.

(a) Specific etiological diagnosis. Technologically advanced communities can hope in the near future to identify most conditions leading to severe retardation. Except possibly for Down syndrome and a few others, the resources of skill, technology, finance and infra-structure are not generally available in developing countries.

(b) A significant degree of permanent cerebral impairment. But what degree, and how is impairment and its significance measured? Intelligence tests are problematic even where developed and standardized, and are of very doubtful trans-cultural validity (Serpell, 1972a, 1972b, 1977). It would be better to ignore permanance since the most important group of children to identify are those who appear retarded but can be treated.

(c) Deviation from developmental norms. Unfortunately, age-related norms are not available for most communities throughout the world and establishing them can be time consuming especially where ages are not normally recorded or recalled. The International Epidemiological Studies of Childhood Disability (I.E.S.C.D.) (Belmont, 1981 and susbsequent workshop reports) are tackling the problems of designing questionnaires which are standardized but accommodate to varying cultural norms of development.

(d) Discordance with expected social roles. The most obvious example is the emergence of mildly retarded children with the spread of effective universal primary education. More severely impaired children are unable to fulfill roles even of self care and may be recognised in any society, even if concepts and perceptions are subject to wide cultural variation (Miles, 1981).

Thus there are many ways of approaching the same problem. In most communities clinical and pathological models are less likely to be relevant and useful than developmental models viewed in the context of specific cultures. It should be remembered that screening may directly identify disorders or merely indicate indirectly the probability of a disorder being present. Probability or risk is a statistical concept, and factors which qualify it locally should be taken into account wherever possible.

3. **Is the procedure safe?** This may be difficult to judge without thorough evaluation, but non-invasive techniques do not usually raise any serious difficulties. When screening in pregnancy, safety of both mother and baby needs to be considered.

4. **Is the procedure acceptable?** This depends on the cultural factors which determine common or general perceptions of the issues, and psychological factors which affect individual perceptions. Thus the information available and the degree of understanding which can be achieved in the community, and the manner in which tests or examinations are offered to individuals are both equally important. Moreover, independent of the specific issues relating to any one screening program, the provenance and general approach of workers to a community will determine the degree to which they are trusted and accepted. The local experience of previous health care interventions must also be taken into account. All this makes it particularly important that screening programs are planned wherever possible within broad primary health care projects.

5. **Does the test discriminate well: Is it reliable?** Reliability is a measure of the consistency of the results of the same procedure with different circumstances of time, place and personnel. It is obtained partly by good test design but also by obtaining trained committed personnel with a good conceptual understanding and the ability to evaluate their own performance. These are conditions difficult to achieve, but inter-observer variation prejudices statistical comparison and cross-cultural value. Many disabilities are only identified in early years by observations of developmental delay which are necessarily age dependent. In many communities personal ages have never been culturally necessary and are not known beyond the first year. Extension of schooling and use of birth certificates is changing this in some places, but in others it may still be necessary to establish a local 'calender of significant events' by which to reckon individual ages. Anthropometric work might eventually help in this field but it is probably better to rely on widely understood procedures such as touching the ear over the head to indicate age over about five years. Without some objective basis, lack of trust or too great a willingness to please may render age data completely unreliable.

6. **Does the test discriminate well: Is it valid?** Validity is concerned with the degree to which the distribution of results of screening correlate with that of the target disorder in the population examined. 'Sensitivity' measures its ability to identify all positive cases and miss none; a very sensitive test gives very few false negatives. 'Specificity' measures its ability to identify all true negative cases and miss none; a very specific test gives few false positives. However, these technical measures are less likely to pose problems than the precise target definition as discussed above. Without a clear and consistent definition it is impossible to know what is a true positive or true negative. With inappropriate definitions plucked from 'western' experience, seeking a valid screening test will be in vain. Pragmatically, a test may be considered valid if it succeeds in picking up many cases in which intervention can be effective. For example in some Zambian communities there can be little doubt that the Campaign failed to reach many children, but those that were discovered represented a valid and valuable beginning to a long term process of development, and possibly as many as could initially be helped.

7. **Can the 'negatives' be reassured?** In situations of low sensitivity, the many children giving false negatives, or their parents, are reassured spuriosly, and reassurance to all is thereby devalued. This is important when the screening detects pre-symptomatic evidence of disease processes, such as the detection of congenital hypothyroidism by the 'blood spot' test, but for serious, overt disability it is barely relevant because children will generally be aware of their own problems.

8. **Is there any risk of harm?** Some ill-effects or risks of application of a screening test may be acceptable to those in whom the target disorder is discovered and who can benefit from the intervention. They are not acceptable to others, who receive no benefit. Many evasive techniques applied in pregnancy tests pose particularly problematic risks to all those subjected to screening. Where initial screening has selected children for further investigation or treatment, the hazards of such intervention may be unacceptable to those falsely thought to be 'positive' but with no prospect of benefit. In screening for disability, such as hearing loss, the worst that is likely to be experienced is inconvenience and unfulfilled expectations.

9. Do we know enough of the natural history of the disorder to evaluate interventions? Without this we cannot know whether or not pre-symptomatic screening and subsequent interventions are justified. With overt disability in older children, such as those with post polio deformities, we can rely upon observable improvements in function, performance, social opportunities and expressed satisfaction. For intellectual impairment, known norms of language development may offer the soundest basis for screening (Clarke & Clarke, 1981). But of course, the 'natural' history of these children, that is, the likely course of events without specific intervention, is a complex web of disadvantage combining biological impairment, educational deprivation, and social stigma and discrimination. Habilitation must address itself to all these elements of handicap.

10. Can we intervene successfully? Unless the progress of disability or its personal and social consequences can be ameliorated and the lives of individuals enhanced by intervention, screening is not justified. This depends upon the logistic as well as technical possibilities, and the availability of resources. Screening programs may need to discriminate between positives, according to the type of intervention required. For example, mentally retarded children must be identified in terms of the potential for recovery. Some will need primarily improved nutrition and treatment; others will need primarily care, education and social support. Built into the Zambian Campaign was a fundamental principle that no child should be identified as disabled without offering some immediate help. This 'provisional care plan' included simple advice to child, family or school, guidance on construction of aids, provision of training documents, encouraging parents, siblings or others to accept rehabilitatory roles and undertake training programs and so on (Fryers, 1983).

Screening type surveys might be justified in terms of improvements for future generations through improved plans for prevention or rehabilitation, but it is probably true that we already know enough to plan such programs in most cases: the problems in developing countries are more commonly associated with implementation. The same principle applies: screening programs are justified by the effectiveness of subsequent interventions.

11. Can we reach the target population? A total community may not need to be subjected to specific screening procedures, or it may not be feasible to do so. Selection of a high risk group might require working through village health care workers, community leaders or the people in general after sufficient and appropriate publicity and education. The Zambian Campaign used a combination of all three, but the I.E.S.C.D. project design was to screen whole populations of children aged 4 to 9 years. It has also piloted screening instruments in a wide variety of different communities, reflecting the problems encountered. Perhaps ideally, instruments should be field tested in the communities chosen for the screening, in a continous process of monitoring and evaluation. Building this into primary health care infra-structure will not be easy but may be the best way of learning relevant skills and improving techniques.

To reach the selected population, all the problems of logistics, communication and acceptance which prejudice delivery will need to be tackled. Access poses many problems, for instance where strangers, especially men, do not normally enter compounds or speak to women. Remote villages with firm traditional authority structures pose different problems from urban communities where there is greater likelihood of contact with the services at birth and school entry.

Communication across cultures is always subtle and complex. Translation into local languages is essential for any written documents used for the screening, but some concepts are not translatable into some languages, and even the aims of the program may not be understandable in some cultures. Local personnel are almost certainly best, but at least workers must have achieved genuine acceptance, trust and respect (see Narayanan, 1981). This should be so in any primary health care setting.

Easier access may inevitably be available to a small, wealthy, educated elite who do not represent the target population, but their involvement may be exploited as a very influential group who represent the aspirations of the people. The intrinsic cohesion of many village communities may lead to whole villages sharing progressive attitudes and economic and social development. Such villages may well lead the way in health care also, and it is quite likely that a better infra-structure and lower child mortality would render them most appropriate to initiate screening programs that others may follow.

12. Is the cost reasonable in the light of probable benefits? There is no easy way to answer this question. Cost benefit analyses are very rare in technologically advanced societies and cannot be readily used in different economic, organizational and cultural contexts. Certainly the question should be taken very seriously before embarking upon any program, and the best assessment possible made with the information available. Moreover, monitoring and evaluation should be built in wherever possible, though again, developed countries have usually neglected this. It is also worth pointing out that treatment programs and procedures should be similarly subjected to cost vetting!

DISABILITY, PRIMARY HEALTH CARE, AND COMMUNITY BASED REHABILITATION

It is clear that screening faces many hazards in developing countries. Problems of communication, access, and logistics are perhaps most obvious, but defining target disorders and target populations, and ensuring valid screening procedures are equally difficult. The greatest problem, and certainly the most important issue in planning any program, is the effectiveness of subsequent interventions and their delivery. It may be acceptable simply to identify children with any overt serious disability if local workers can tailor rehabilitation to their individual needs, but the most sophisticated classification of disorders will be wasted if children identified receive no help.

In communities with comprehensive primary school provision, it may be feasible to screen all children at school entry, but even there, many disabled children are likely not to be in school. Where there is skilled monitoring and recording at childbirth, it may be possible to follow up a cohort of children, monitoring them for both illness and developmental delay, instituting habilitation programs as required, and providing usually unavailable demographic data (Fryers, 1981).

It seems obvious that such programs should be part of primary health care, but recent important writings on P.H.C., whilst properly emphasizing prevention of, for example, polio, barely acknowledge the problems of children already disabled (e.g. Morley, Rhode, & Williams, 1983). Yet quite apart from present need throughout the world, as infant mortality is reduced we may well see an increase in survival of children with some types of serious impairment. The 'illness' model which has dominated medical thinking in all countries seems to have difficulty in accommodating permanent impairment not subject to 'treatment' even where every effort is made to fit it to the cultures of developing countries (Bennett, 1979). Similarly, educational thinking almost everywhere has been dominated by specialist and separatist models of provision for children with special education needs.

Development of special medical and educational facilities are likely to be very limited by cost, and to be available largely to an urban elite, but in any case this is unlikely to be the best. In most developing countries there is a strong movement away from separate facilities which are necessarily stigmatizing and alienating, and developing communities have a chance of something much better from the start (Heron & Myers, 1983). Community-based rehabilitation aims to provide local help to disabled people to live lives as normal as possible within their own families, to enjoy a normal range of relationships, to participate in activities and opportunities valued in their own culture, and to contribute positively to their community. Generally, people of all ages will best learn appropriate personal and social skills in the community where they will use them, and all communities have resources to forward that learning process. They also have resources for providing much practical help such as physical aids.

The identification and mobilization of these resources is one important task for local community workers, but those engaged currently in primary education or health care may well need extra training to enable them to do this. The WHO manual *Training the Disabled in the Community* (Helander et al., 1980) is an attempt at providing comprehensive training packages for community workers or others such as parents to use. UNICEF and Rehabilitation International have produced a more compact document. Practical help in making aids, for example to allow a child to sit up, observe his surroundings and communicate with people instead of lying on the ground, is available (e.g. from AHRTAG, 1980), and there is much useful advice in some widely available publications (e.g. Werner 1976, 1977; King, King, & Martodipoero, 1978). For severely retarded children this is discussed in more detail elsewhere (Fryers, 1984, chapter 14).

Local workers will also need supervision and support within an adequate infra-structure. One of the most important needs is an enlarged repertory of ideas for what can be done for disabled children within the resources of the village community. Local registers of disabled children may help in the organization and monitoring of rehabilitation for all those in need but should be kept simple. Local experience may produce invaluable information for regional or national planning. For example, the Zambia Campaign has stimulated new thinking on the possibilities of cheap locally produced spectacles and other developments (Parekh & Serpell, 1983).

Perhaps the most important thing in all this is to find ways of promoting positive attitudes toward disabled children. They can be helped; they can get more satisfaction in life; they can be contributors. The most effective way is to demonstrate it and it is hoped that projects and programs now in operation will be able to do this (e.g. Rao, 1983). We need more examples of effective action on behalf of disabled children; only then can we be confident that screening, early case finding and monitoring will be worthwhile.

References

AHRTAG (1980). *Playing together: Aids for disabled children.* London: Appropriate Health Resources and Technologies Action Group Ltd.

Belmont, L. (Ed.) (1981). Severe mental retardation across the world: Epidemiological studies. *International Journal of Mental Health, 10*(1).

Bennett, F. J. (1979). *Community diagnosis and health action.* London: MacMillan.

Clarke, A. M. & Clarke, A. D. B. (1981). Problems of applying behavioral measures in assessing incidence and prevalence of severe mental retardation in developing countries. *International Journal of Mental Health, 10*(1), 76-84.

Fryers, T. (1981). Problems in screening for mental retardation in developing countries. *International Journal of Mental Health, 10*(1), 64-75.

Fryers, T. (1983). *Report on initial evaluation of the Zambia National Campaign to Reach Disabled Children.* Lusaka: Ministry of Education.

Fryers, T. (1984). *The epidemiology of severe intellectual impairment: The dynamics of prevalence.* London: Academic Press.

Hammerman, S. & Maikowski, S. (1981). *The economics of disability: International perspectives.* New York: Rehabilitation International/United Nations.

Helander, E., Mendis, P., & Nelson, G. (1980). *Training the disabled in the community: An experimental manual on rehabilitation and disability prevention for developing countries.* Geneva: World Health Organization.

Heron, A. & Myers, M. (1983). *Intellectual impairment: The battle against handicap.* London: Academic Press.

King, M., King, F., & Martodipoero, S. (1978). *Primary child care: A manual for health workers.* Oxford: O.U.P.

Miles, M. (1981). *A survey of handicapped children and their needs in the North West Frontier Province (of Pakistan).* Peshawar: Mission Hospital Mental Health Center.

Morley, D., Rhode, J., & Williams, G. (1983). *Practising health for all.* Oxford: O.U.P.

Narayanan, H. S. (1981). A study of prevalence of mental retardation in Southern India. *International Journal of Mental Health, 10*(1), 28-36.

Ng'andu, S. K. & Sinyangwe, I. M. (1981). *Final report of the feasibility study for Zambia National Campaign to Reach Disabled Children.* Lusaka: University of Zambia Educational Research Bureau.

Parekh, P. K. & Serpell, R. (1983). *Report of national planning seminar on the rationale and logistics of specialist intervention in relation to community based rehabilitation.* Lusaka: IYDP Commission.

Paul, F. M. (1981). The problems of mental subnormality in a developing country. In P. Mittler (Ed.), *Frontiers of knowledge in mental retardation.* Baltimore: University Park Press.

Rao, A. (1983). *Community based intervention for disabled children: Experiences and insights.* New Delhi: UNICEF.

Serpell, R. (1972a). Intelligence tests in the third world. *Race Today, 4*, 2.

Serpell, R. (1972b). How perception differs among cultures. *New Society, June*, 619-623.

Serpell, R. (1977). Estimates of intelligence in a rural community of Eastern Zambia. In F. M. Oktacha (Ed.), *Modern psychology and cultural adaptation.* Nairobi: Swahili Language Cons. & Publications.

Stein, Z. (1981). Why is it useful to measure incidence and prevalence? *International Journal of Mental Health, 10*(1), 14-22.

Werner, D. B. (1976). *Health care and human dignity: Proceedings of a symposium on appropriate technology and delivery of health and welfare services for the disabled in developing countries.* London: Coomonwealth Foundation (Occasional Paper XLI).

Werner, D. B. (1977). *Where there is no doctor.* Palo Alto: Hesperian Foundation.

WHO (1980). *International classification of impairments, disabilities, and handicaps.* Geneva: World Health Organization.

3

CEREBRAL PALSY: ISSUES IN INCIDENCE, EARLY DETECTION, AND HABILITATION IN PORTUGAL

Maria da Graça de Campos Andrada

Cerebral palsy is the most frequent motor disability in childhood. It is not a well defined and clear situation but a complex and heterogenous clinical picture with different syndromes and disabilities. The etiology is also usually multiple and frequently not very clear due to the interaction of adverse prenatal, perinatal, and postnatal problems. The common factor in all cerebral palsy syndromes is the existence of a neurodevelopmental disability affecting several areas of child development and creating specific problems regarding the child's habilitation.

We can define cerebral palsy as a clinical syndrome resulting from a static cerebral lesion which is affected by and interferes with the process of brain maturation and development. It occurs early in the child's life due to adverse prenatal, perinatal, and postnatal problems. It is not an hereditary disease but in some cases a genetic predisposing factor may be present. Prenatal factors are considered when the child is S.F.D. (small for gestational age) or when we detect abnormalities during pregnancy, such as bleeding, placental anomalies, eclampsia, diabetes, or infection of the fetus.

Strongly indicating prenatal factors or the possibility of a genetic syndrome or chromosomic anomaly is the finding of dysmorphic traits or malformations during the physical examination of the child. When this happens, we must be careful of genetic counseling, since what it actually involved may be a genetic syndrome with neurological signs.

Perinatal factors are considered when obvious abnormalities occur just before, during, or after birth (first week of life). The most important in this group is anoxia, responsible for the lesion in about 40 to 50 percent of cases. Hyperbilirubinemia is a decreasing factor but unfortunately one still responsible for some of our cases, due to deficient perinatal assistance. The association of hyperbilirubinemia and anoxia has proved to be more dangerous in the incidence of brain lesion, and as reported by Hagberg (1975), S.F.D. babies are particularly sensitive to these factors. This association is an example of the interaction of adverse factors frequently responsible for the pathogenesis of cerebral palsy. Multiple pregnancy, prolonged, and/or difficult labour are also adverse factors. Pelvic delivery, if not adequately managed by cesarian section, is frequently associated with cerebral palsy.

It is a well known fact that periventricular hemorrhage in the premature baby is a frequent cause of death. If the baby survives—the lesion not being severe—the clinical picture of spastic diplegia is commonly present with more involvement of the lower limb fibers of the spinal tract. Hypoglycemia, sepsis, meningitis, or dehydration in the early newborn period are also adverse factors that may produce brain lesions.

Postnatal factors are considered when brain damage occurs between the seventh day of life and two years of age. The damage may be due to to infections of the central nervous system, such as meningitis, encephalitis, tumour, hydrocephalus, etc., or to hydroelectrolytic disturbances in early life.

In approximately 20% of the cases the etiology of cerebral palsy is unknown. The relative incidence of the different etiologies varies according to the state of health care in each country, and so does the clinical picture and degree of accompanying motor disability and/or mental retardation.

In 1979 a retrospective study done at our Center of 2,259 children with cerebral palsy showed a very high incidence of perinatal causes. The distribution of cases according to birth date did not show much improvement with the years (Figure 1). The incidence of cerebral palsy is always higher in males. In our statistics, 57.8% of those with the condition were boys and 42.2% were girls.

The child with cerebral palsy always has a sensorimotor disability, which consists mainly of a disturbance of tonus and posture, with abnormal patterns of movement, persistent and pathological reflex postures, and delayed acquisition of normal postural reactions necessary to overcome the force of gravity and to allow the child normal sensorimotor experiences that are so important for developing the basic skills essential for more complex activities.

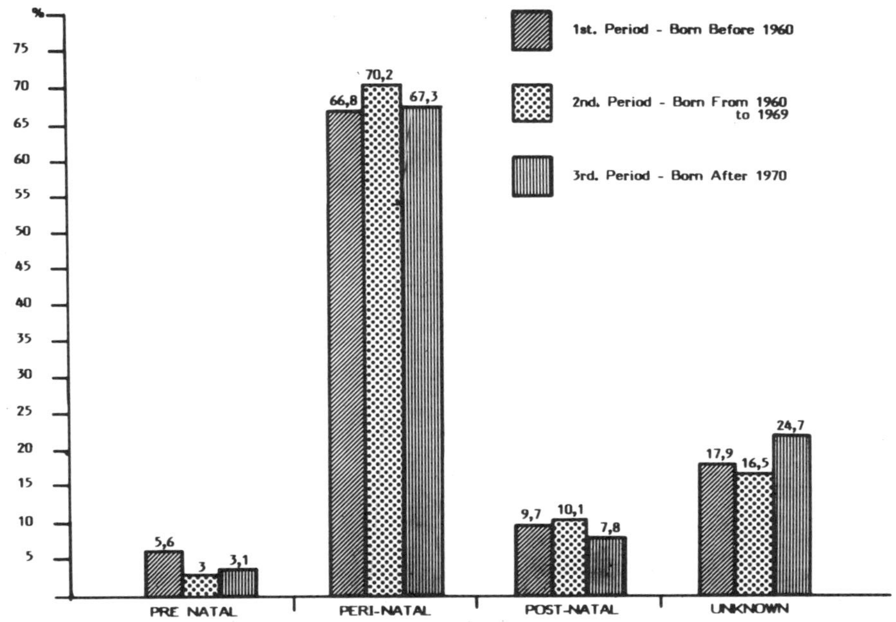

Figure 1. Comparison of Types of Etiology Over Three Periods

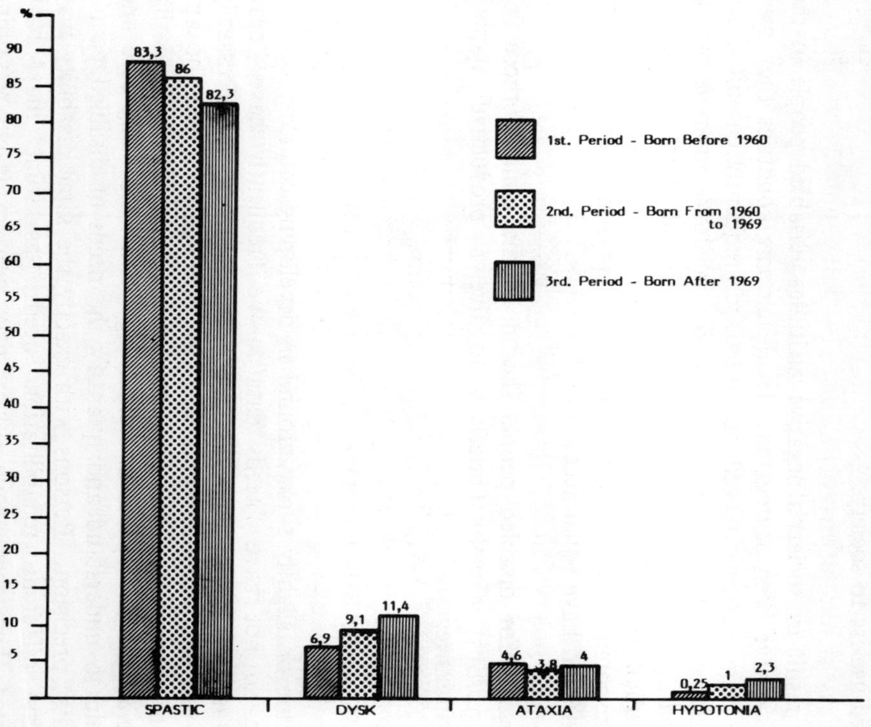

Figure 2. Clinical Types and Their Incidence Over Three Periods

There are different clinical syndromes related to different areas of central nervous system involvement which are also related in some way to the type and degree of brain injury. The spastic syndromes are the most frequent—85.5% of all cases (Figure 2). These include:

- the spastic hemiplegias with only one side of the body affected;
- the spastic diplegias in which the lower limbs are more and symmetrically affected and the upper limbs are minimally and usually asymmetrically involved;
- the spastic tetraplegias with the four limbs equally involved or with greater involvement in the upper extremeties.

These spastic tetraplegias are frequently mixed with other neurological signs, like athetosis, dystonia, and/or ataxia. Many of these cases have suprabulbar paresis with speech impairment. They are frequently asymmetrical and some authors, like Ingram (1964, 1965), include them in a separate group of double hemiplegias.

The dyskinetic syndromes present in our group of children in 9.2% of cases include athetosis, coreoathetosis, and dystonia. In all three situations, there are involuntary movements and changing tonus; however, while in athetosis and coreoathetosis the basic tonus is usually low and the prognosis regarding function is better, in dystonic syndrome there is a basic hypertonus with marked changes and severe abnormal postures which interfere greatly with function.

The ataxic syndrome present in 4.1% of our cases includes the clinical picture of ataxia with motor incoordination, disturbances in equilibrium (disequilibrium syndrome), and ataxic diplegia, with ataxia and mild spasticity in the lower limbs. The remaining percentage of our cases (1.2%) show hypotonia and are usually cases in which the diagnosis is not yet clear due to young age of the child, or to minor neurologic dysfunction.

The child with cerebral palsy may have, as we have seen, different types of neuromotor impairments and different degrees of motor disability which interfere with function and experiences, but there are many other disabilities as well. Visual problems are frequent and may include strabismus, refractive errors, optic atrophy, or visual field defects. Hearing loss is more common when the cause is hyperbilirubinemia or anoxia due to lesion of the cochlear nerve or auditory nuclei, and is usually associated with the dyskinetic syndromes. The loss is usually a partial one present only in the high frequencies; therefore, sometimes the loss is not detected early, if not investigated carefully. It affects speech since consonants (high frequency sounds) are very important for speech comprehension.

Speech is also affected by other problems in cerebral palsy. The most important and frequent speech defect is dysarthria which is caused by motor dysfunction of the speech organs. It is more frequent in dyskinetic syndromes and also in many cases of tetraplegias, mainly the mixed forms with suprabulbar paresis. Developmental aphasia may also be present. Many children have language and speech delay due to mental retardation which is usually present in about 50% of cases.

In our own data 21.7% of the children we examined showed normal intelligence, and in the groups divided according to the year of birth (Figure 3), we found a mild improvement in level of mental functioning over the years; an increasing number of children showed normal intelligence while there was a reduction in the percentage of children with severe mental retardation. However, in children born after 1960, we found 38.8% of children with severe mental retardation. The limitations these children have in early sensorimotor experiences, and the difficulties in communication they show make their evaluation difficult with regard to cognitive competence; consequently, early and continuous assessment and guidance are very essential.

Many children have perceptual difficulties which interfere with their learning to read and write; the motor dysfunction and communication problems also frequently interfere with children's learning. Since convulsions might complicate the clinical picture, antiepileptic treatment is recommended. Cases with epilepsy usually have more unclear prognosis.

EARLY DETECTION AND PREVENTION: IMPORTANCE OF BRAIN PLASTICITY AND RISK FACTORS

Some impairments are present and can be detected at birth, but as is generally the case in cerebral palsy, most of the problems, although present at birth, become obvious only as the child grows and develops. Since cognitive competence increases during maturation as stimuli and experiences provided by the environment mould the developing brain, we can well understand the importance of the early detection of disability. The presence of a so called developmental disability in a child may disturb not only cognitive competence as a whole but also such other functions as mobility, perception, speech and behavior, or emotional adjustment. Early stimulation is

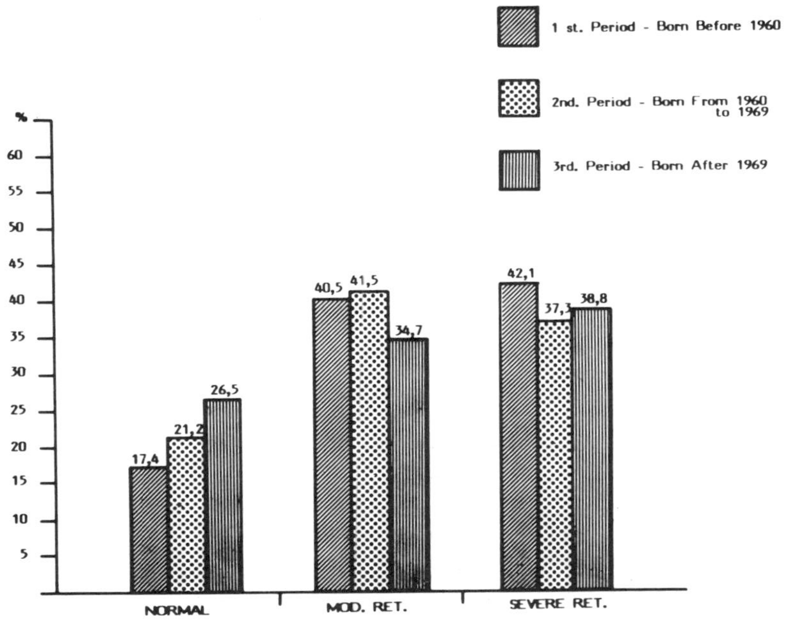

Figure 3. Comparison of Mental Levels Over Three Periods

necessary if the child is to overcome these difficulties.

As we know, there is limited potential for regeneration after a brain lesion, but it seems that the same activity can be performed in several different ways. Brain plasticity is assumed to be much greater in early life than in later life, as can be shown by the easier recovery from acquired child aphasia compared to recovery from acquired aphasia in adults. Although there already is some hemispheric asymmetry and specialization during the early developmental stages, reorganization of genetically predisposed pathways seems to be possible.

Recovery from brain lesions may be explained by various mechanisms. In the acute stages, early recovery probably reflects disappearance of brain swelling and/or of temporary dysfunction around the lesion, resorption of hemorrhages, improvement of vascular perfusion, and regression of transient metabolic disturbances. It may also reflect recovery from synaptic dysfunction. This is a spontaneous process mainly influenced by a good general condition of the child and is not due to any specific stimulation. We frequently find signs of irritability and/or convulsions, as well as some neurological signs in newborn babies that may disappear and have no significance, or become more marked and represent signs of brain lesion.

Late recovery is more difficult to explain, but it might reflect the organization of brain function and structure with new synapses and new pathways. This might be the result of regrowth of axons that are able to reoccupy the vacated myelin sheaths due to lesion or synaptic remodeling. We do not know the extent to which this happens in human beings, but evidence exists in fetal monkeys (Goldman & Rakic, 1981) of the proliferation of fibres even to the other hemisphere after a focal lesion, a finding which underscores the importance of interhemispheric commissures. Evidence also exists of the growth of axons in the hypocampus of the rat. Spinelli, Jansen, and Viana di Risco (1980) also demonstrated that in kittens between 4 and 10 weeks of age, training the foreleg to move in order to avoid an electric shock was associated with a 30% increase in the basal dendrites of pyramidal cells in the sensorimotor cortex. This increase was no longer possible after the 10th week of life.

The importance of specific stimulation and of the timing of these stimuli has been underscored in several animal experiments reviewed by Prechtl (1981). These studies revealed the presence and later disappearance of transient neuronal structures—mainly synapses in the brain—during a limited period of time. As Prechtl mentions, function may play a prominent role in epigenetic shaping of the neural structure, although the extent seems rather limited and the time of effective influence restricted to relatively short critical periods.

Another mechanism for recovery of function is a more active use of alternate potentially usable, but still subsidiary, pathways to achieve the same goal or of different strategies to stimulate the system. Examples of such strategies are sign language and the Bliss System which have proved to be good methods for improving the acquisition of language. All these important aspects of brain plasticity and environmental factors, able to shape the neuronal structures, even if only for a short period in early life, stress the importance of early detection of a child's handicap and of early stimulation along neurodevelopmental lines.

Also deserving emphasis is the importance of early mother-child interaction, so frequently disturbed when the child has a handicap. The importance of play in the child's development is similarly notable. The handling of the child to improve sensorimotor experiences is a very important method of helping brain maturation. The impotance of limbic commissure and affective stimuli in the early stages of development is well recognized. Thus early detection and management should be based upon two important points:

- preserve the mother-child interaction process, avoiding worries;
- involve the parents in the handling of the child so that they may learn how to find their child's potentialities and relate as normally as possible to their child.

With regard to the first point, it is important to consider the following caveat: Although we should explain to parents the problems they have to face, since prognosis is usually difficult in the early stages, we should avoid terms such as brain lesion and mental deficiency; instead, we should speak about developmental disability, brain dysfunction, or slowness.

We always prefer to talk about handling instead of "treatment" in order to avoid medicalization and to ensure that parents regard their child not as a handicapped child but as a child with a handicap. We should "treat" or handle the child when we find abnormal patterns of postures that disturb the child's development, but should also be able to recognize such normal variations in children as the developmental delay of the premature, differences between neurological signs of immaturity and lesion, and normal variations of tonus and primitive reflexes.

The difference between normality and abnormality is not sharp. Thus when manipulated with stress postures, many children can simulate abnormal patterns regarded as pathological on a first assessment and as normal a few weeks later. Evidence corroborating this observation exists in data we collected. Frequently the signs of immaturity subside and the child becomes normal. Touwen (1976) has also presented evidence of great variations in primitive reflexes in normal children, and so the persistence of some reflexes may be a normal variation in child development. Diagnosis requires a great deal of experience in evaluating child neurodevelopmental disabilities if false diagnosis or misdiagnosis of affected children is to be avoided. When we are not sure about a suspected handicap, it is better to examine the child again within two weeks or a month rather than unnecessarily upsetting the parents.

Early detection is also a preventive strategy not only because it may help to avoid secondary disabilities but also because it may be a way to call attention to the main causes and thereby lead to improved perinatal care. Hagberg (1979) has demonstrated the correlation between decrease in perinatal mortality, due to improved perinatal care, and the incidence of cerebral palsy. He reports not only decrease in number but also improvement in the quality of life as reflected by a much less incidence of severe neurological syndromes.

In a 1979 survey of all children observed in our Centre since 1960, we compared children's development over the years and came to the following conclusions:

- perinatal risk in Portugal was still very high, with a very high incidence of avoidable neurological handicaps;
- in the great majority of cases, the degree of the handicaps was severe, with high incidence of spastic or mixed types of tetraplegia and mental retardation;
- there was improvement only in the degree of mental retardation—there was a higher incidence of children with normal intelligence in the last five years of the period studied; and
- the degree of motor handicap did not show any improvement over the years (Andrada, 1979; Andrada, Guerreiro, & Ramos da Costa, 1980).

On the basis of our findings we stressed the need to improve perinatal care and early detection, calling attention to the adverse risk factors.

Perinatal mortality in this country, although on the decline, is still very high compared with the rate in Sweden for example (see Figure 4). We do not know the incidence of cerebral palsy in Portugal, but judging from the correlation between perinatal mortality and the incidence of cerebral palsy reported by Hagberg in an epidemiological study done in Sweden, we can estimate an incidence rate of about 2% of births. This figure corresponds to the figures for Sweden in the sixties (Hagberg, Hagberg, & Olow, 1975a, 1975b, 1976). In a recent survey of the children evaluated at the Calouste Gulbenkian Center in 1983, we found that although there has been some improvement in early detection, we still receive only 35.5% of the cases before one year of age. This percentage includes children evaluated in our developmental assessment clinic for risk babies born in the University Hospital and treated in the Intensive Care Unit. During the period 1970-79 26.6% of cases were seen before one year of age.

There has, however, been a significant decrease in the percentage of children born at home in comparison with 1979 statistics. From 1970 to 1979, 11,8% of the cases were born at home. Among the cases we examined in 1983, 2.72% of those born before 1979 were born at home compared to 1.8% for children born at home after 1979. The situation regarding children with cerebral palsy detected in our Risk Baby Clinic has not improved since 1979; the data in Table 1 show a higher incidence in 1980 and 1982.

The developmental problems found in our Risk Baby Clinic for children born in 1982 are reported in Table 2. The total number of births in Portugal was 151,029 in 1982. From the 294 children examined, the children born in the University Hospital showed the lowest incidence of neurological handicaps, followed by children born in the local hospital, children born in private maternity facilities, and finally children born at home (Andrada, 1982). Although these figures may not be completely significant due to the small number of home-birth children examined—only 2—we believe this seems to reflect the real picture of the situation in the country. Even private maternity facilities frequently create problems for the newborn because they lack good pediatric perinatal assistance. The risk factors responsible for the 19 cases of neurological handicaps found in this group are reported in Table 3. In many cases several risk factors interfered, sometimes one facilitating the others.

The importance of the following risk factors associated with the incidence of cerebral palsy needs to be stressed: mild anoxia (3.9%); severe anoxia (10.1%); pelvic delivery (11.1%); low birth weight for

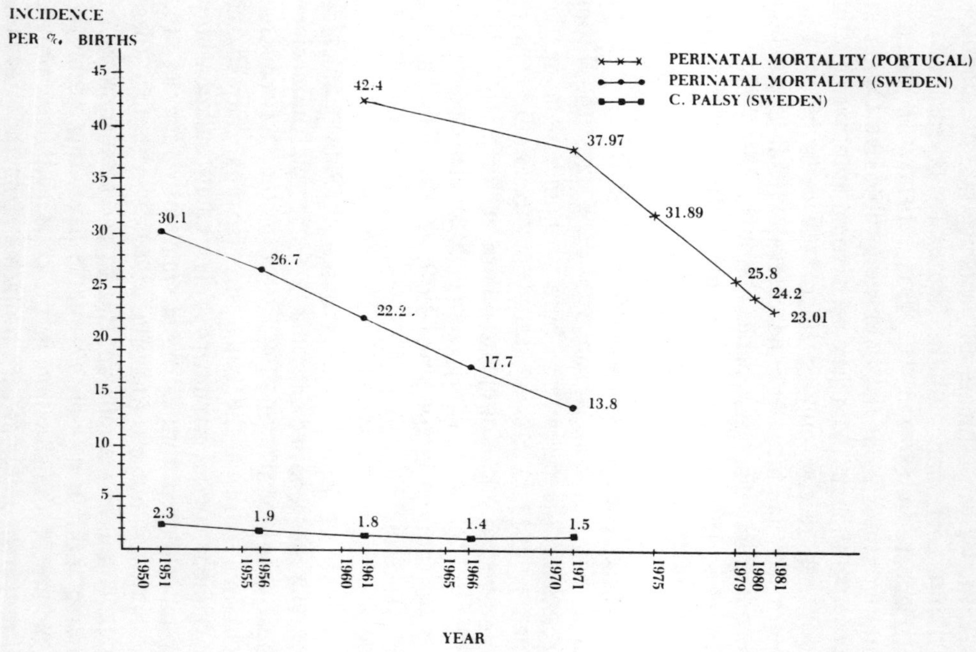

Figure 4. Perinatal Mortality and Cerebral Palsy: Portugal and Sweden

Table 1. Risk Babies Born at the University Hospital

Year	Number of Births	Number of Children Examined	Diagnosis: C.Palsy		Diagnosis: Psyco-Motor Retardation		Total Afected Cases	
1976	2675	103	9	(3,3 ‰)	8	(3,0 ‰)	17	(6,3 ‰)
1977	2843	234	11	(3,8 ‰)	6	(2,1 ‰)	17	(5,9 ‰)
1978	2942	269	7	(2,3 ‰)	5	(1,7 ‰)	12	(4,0 ‰)
1979	3082	216	6	(1,9 ‰)	6	(1,9 ‰)	12	(3,8 ‰)
1980	3265	304	7	(2,1 ‰)	5	(1,5 ‰)	12	(3,6 ‰)
1981								
1982	2815	228	7	(2,5 ‰)	4	(1,4 ‰)	11	(3,9 ‰)

Table 2. Developmental Problems Among 294 Cases Born 1982

Diagnosis	Place of Birth: Central Hosp. or Mat.	Local Hosp.	Private Mat	Home
Normal Devel.	210	16	25	1
Palpebral Ptosis	2 (Forceps)			
Cong. Torticolis	2			
Facial Palsy	3 (Forceps)			
Braquial Palsy	2			
Vision Defect	3		2	
Strabismus	1			
Cong.Club Feet	1			
Cong. Myopathy	1 (Myot.Dist)			
Genetic Synd	2	2	1(Chrom.an.)	
Psychomotor Retard and Epilepsy	6 2,5%	1 5%		
Cerebral Palsy	7 3,4%	1 5%	3 9,4%	1 50%
Total	240	20	32	2

Table 3. Risk Factors Associated With 19 Affected of 294 Cases

Etiological Factors	Registered	Afected	%
Cong. Cadiopathy Surgery Comp.	1	1	100%
Pre Eclampsia	14	1	7,1%
Multiple Pregnancy	23	1	4,3%
Placental Anomalies	2	1	50%
Diabetes	15	1	6,6%
Pelvic Delivery	18	2	11,1%
Forceps	37	2	5,4%
Cesarian	60	4	6,6%
Hiperbilirrubinemia	44	1 *	2,2%
S.F.D.	22	4	18,1%
Prematurity B.W. > 1000gr G.A. > 28 Sem	48	2	4,2%
Extreme Imaturity B.W. < 1000gr G.A. < 28 S	4	0	0%
Severe Anoxia (Apgar 1m 0-3)	79	8	10,1%
Mod. or Mild Anoxia (Apgar 1m 4-7)	76	3	3,9%
R.D.S.	8	1 **	11,1%
Cong.Infections	4 ***	2	50%
Perinatal Infection (Sepsis)	2	0	0%

* S.F.D. + Anoxia + Ict

** Pneumotorax

*** 2 Unknown Etiology; 1 Tox, 1 Rubella

Table 4. Pathological Cases—Assessment Clinic

Condition	Cases		
Cerebral Palsy	110	58.8%	
		Mild	1 case
		Moderate	4 cases
Mental Retardation	13	Profound	3 cases
		Undet.	5 cases
Familiar microcephaly	1		
Brain Malformation	1		
Arrested Hydrocephalus	1		
Meningo Encephalitis sequelae	1		
Heredo Degen. Brain Dys.	5		
Chromosomal Anomalies	1		
Rubella Embryopathy	3		
Other Empbryopathies	1		
Genetic Syndromes	2		
Epilepsy	5		
Developmental Aphasia	1		
Minimal Brain Dys.	5		
Infantile Autism	1		
Behavior Disorders	2		
Strabismus	1		
Hearing Deficiency	3		
Neuromuscular Diseases	3		
Without any illness	6		
Total	184		

gestational age (18.1%); congenital infections (50%); placental abnormalities (50%); and congenital heart malformation (complications after surgery—100%).

We still had one case of hyperbilirubinemia (2.2%) who was born at home and afterwards transferred to a local hospital and finally to an intensive care unit, but too late in fact. This illustrates one of the problems we are confronted with in our country where sometimes we have good but delayed assistance—enough to save the life but not the quality of it.

In the group of children already referred to our Clinic in 1983 as being pathological, we had 110 cases of cerebral palsy (58.8%). The incidence of the developmental disabilities evaluated in this group is shown in Table 4. Regarding the 110 cases of cerebral palsy evaluated, we found a high incidence of spastic tetraparesis, many of the cases having mental retardation and poor prognosis. There has been no improvement in the severity of clinical types since 1979, and the main etiological factor in these cases is perinatal anoxia. Many of these cases could be prevented with better perinatal assistance which should be a priority in a developing country such as ours. The right to be born safe, in security, and wanted should be a rule and a priority in every country.

EARLY HABILITATION PROGRAM WITH PARENTAL GUIDANCE AND SUPPORT

If early detection is our goal, we need interdisciplinary teams able to deal with the handicapped child and his family so that we can prevent further disability, help child development, and make possible total integration of the child into the family, school, and community. In our experience, perents of handicapped children in this country—a country with long religious traditions—frequently show guilt complexes. They want the best care for their children, and some do believe in the miracle of cure. They usually blame us—health staff and doctors, mainly—for being unable to prevent their misfortune and for knowing nothing about disability.

Unfortunately they are often right; doctors and health professionals are more aware of acute health situations and hospital care and have very little knowledge of handicapping conditions and chronic illnesses. We need experienced interdisciplinary teams to deal with the handicapped children and their families so that the latter may feel confident. Otherwise, they will look around for different types of advice and oftentimes try expensive miraculous medication or some other methods of "treatment."

Early detection is the only way to give parents confidence in the health services. We have found that parents of a young baby whose condition is detected and helped early are much better able to cope with the problem than when they come to us later after searching around and listening to different and controversial opinions, most of which may be wrong. This wandering from one practitioner to another is due to lack of awareness and knowledge among doctors and

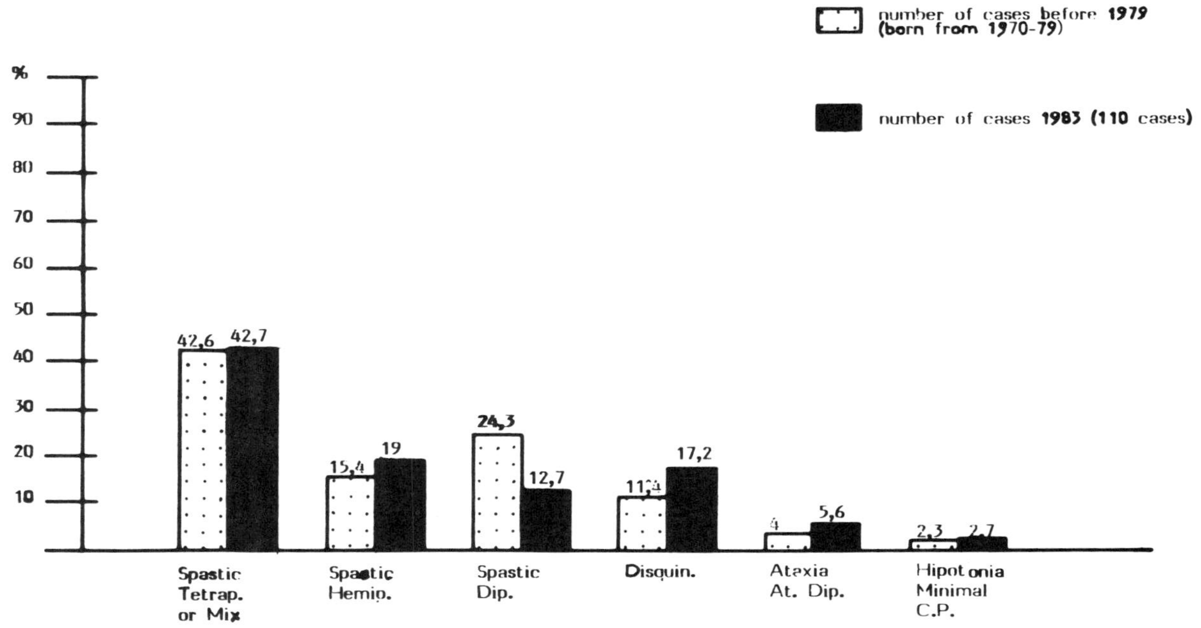

Figure 5. Clinical Types: Comparison of Two Periods

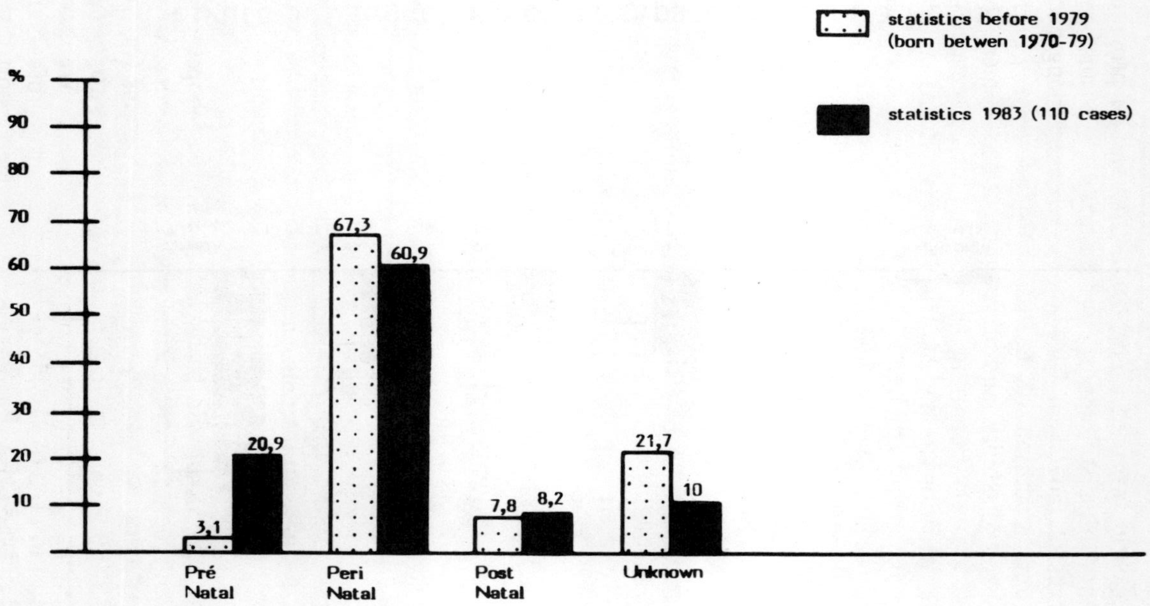

Peri-Natal	Anoxia -	44 cases	40%
	Prematurity -	13 cases	11,8%
	Hiperbilirubinemia -	5 cases	4,5%

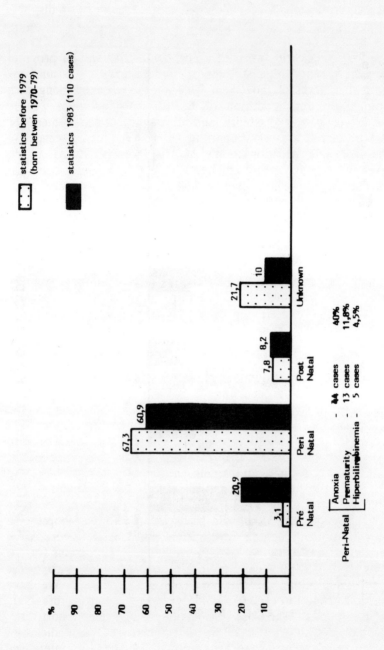

Figure 6. Etiology: Comparison of Two Periods

other health professionals of childhood neurodevelopmental disabilities.

When we detect early, we need a continuous habilitation program with adequate parental interest, support, and guidance. We must develop normal patterns of movement for the affected child along with early stimulation and repetition of normal baby activities. Early detection of childhood disability and developmental assessment of children born at risk are very important ways of improving preventive measures by calling attention to the adverse factors involved, but it also leaves us with too many children and parents needing help and care. In our Center we have had to deal with "early detection" children who always need early treatment, and with the long waiting list of children referred to us by hospitals, health centers, and private pediatricians.

The program of "treatment" must be integrated into the child's normal daily activites if it is to be effective because children learn by repetition. This principle is not easy to communicate to parents because they usually prefer to have the therapist treat the child, performing several exercises once or twice a day, or prescribing medication.

A handicapped child always generates a handicapped family; the child should be part of the family but not the main center of attention. Frequently, in our culture the mother is the only person taking close care of the child during the first year of life. If the child has a handicap, this care lasts through the years. There is the need to involve both parents so that they can help and support each other. We should also bring in grandparents, brothers, and sisters to help and learn about the child's needs and the methods of handling.

The habilitation program should be organized in strict cooperation with the educational programs for children with special needs. Since the beginning of our work, we have been involved in programs for the integration of handicapped children into ordinary school environments and in providing support for special education teachers. We have been getting a great deal of feedback from the educational professionals that we support. When our habilitation staff go to support disabled children in school settings they detect many other handicapped children, never before evaluated, who need the advice of an interdisciplinary team.

How have we been dealing with all these problems? How can we improve early detection and treatment in a country like ours and many other developing countries? We lack adequate facilities and the few existing facilities are still being duplicated by parallel systems of assistance for handicapped children. Through the Association for Cerebral Palsy (APPC), while learning from parents and their needs, we have developed decentralized groups of action involving health and educational professionals, as well as parents and local authorities, to work in programs for early detection, prevention, assistance, and integration. We have learned from previous experiences and we adapt our knowledge to local facilities avoiding duplications and trying to involve the government in this process. This action has been spreading all over the country, first on a regional basis—Lisbon, Coimbra, Porto—and lately at the district level.

As for training of professional teams, we have been organizing courses for doctors in normal child development to prepare them in methods of early detection and to make them aware of neurodevelopmental disabilities during the infancy and early childhood years. We also have been organizing neurodevelopmental courses to prepare therapists already working with handicapped children in children's rehabilitation centers and developmental assessment units.

We have always worked in close association with the Division of Special Education (Ministry of Education) in trying to obtain coordinated action for early detection and treatment, early integration and stimulation with home visiting, and school visiting and advice. Our teams are working more and more outside our center and on the basis of the principle of integration and normalization without forgetting the child's individual special needs and the importance of parental guidance and support.

As noted previously, early management by a competent team gives parents confidence and security so that they are able to discover their child's potentialities and accept the limitations imposed by the disability. But there are frequent crises of disappointment and insecurity which can only be dealt with if there is time to listen to parents and the capacity to make them feel secure. With too many children coming for assessment and guidance, this becomes unbearable as there is no time for reassessment and team discussion involving the parents in decisions to be taken.

Childhood habilitation or rehabilitation is a long and continuous process that should start early and go hand in hand with education.

Health and education are both important to the child; they influence each other throughout the child's life. They must be linked in the care of every child, even more so in the care of the child with a disability.

In early detection and assessment of a child with a handicap, it is impossible for one professional alone to assure and be responsible for identification and treatment, as well as parental guidance and support. Interdisciplinary teams and specialized units are essential, but there is a need for a *key person*, the professional, to be principally responsible and involved in the process according to the nature of the situation.

To improve the child's development, parents as well as the health and educational staff should be prepared to deal with any deviation and special needs in the different areas—health, cognition, emotional, and social. The family of a handicapped child is seeking guidance and support that can only be achieved by the family's involvement in the child's rehabilitation process.

Coordinated habilitation or rehabilitation implies responsibility for all types of handicaps—mental, motor, visual and hearing impairment, multihandicaps, etc. Accordingly, the need for specialized centers with interdisciplinary teams is obvious. Doctors, nurses, and therapists should be trained to function effectively in the area of developmental disabilities. We need pediatric rehabilitation doctors with specific training and adequate curriculum that should include the following: training in pediatrics, child development, and child neurology; and training in rehabilitation pediatrics with emphasis in neurodevelopmental assessment and treatment techniques. Therapists also need to have post-graduate training in these techniques and in child development. Team work with psychologists, social workers, and teachers with an interdisciplinary on-going learning process is a very important way to mutually improve knowledge and assure better assessment and treatment of each child.

Specialized centers should be set up at both regional and district levels located in or in close connection with pediatric hospital units for special diagnostic techniques. These centers should be involved in training programs for doctors and health education personnel in order to improve early detection and provide better care for the handicapped child. Finally, the Center should also be in contact with the primary health care centers involved in early detection and should serve as a resource facility for consultation and advise.

References

Andrada, M. G. (1979). *Epidemiologie des handicaps neurologiques chroniques au Portugal 1979.* Simpósio sobre Prevençao dos Handicaps Neurológicos Crónicos da Criança.

Andrada, M. G. (1982). Diagnóstico da paralisia cerebral-Detecçao e orientaçap precoces. *Revista Portugesa de Pediatria, 13,* 3a.

Andrada, M. G., Guerreiro, O., & Ramos da Costa, M. (1980). Avaliaçao do desenvolvimento da criança em alto risco para deteçao precoce de deficência na infância. *Revista do Desenvolvimento da Criança, 1/2,* 38-41.

Goldman, J. & Rakic, P. C. (1981). Development and plasticity of primate frontal association cortex. In F. O. Schmitt, F. G. Warren, G. Adelman, & S. G. Dennis (Eds.), *The organization of the cerebral cortex.* (pp. 69-97). Cambridge: MIT Press.

Hagberg, B. (1975). Pre, peri, and post natal prevention of major neuropediatric handicaps. *Neuropediatrie, II*(4), 131-338.

Hagberg, B. (1979). Epidemiological and preventive aspects of cerebral palsy and severe mental retardation in Sweden. *European Journal of Pediatrics, 130,* 71-78.

Hagberg, B., Hagberg, G., & Olow, I. (1975a). The changing panorama of cerebral palsy in Sweden—1954-1970: I. Analysis of the general changes. *Acta Pediatrica Scandinavica, 64,* 187-192.

Hagberg, B., Hagberg, G., & Olow, I. (1975b). The changing panorama of cerebral palsy in Sweden—1954-1970: II. Analysis of various syndromes. *Acta Pediatrica Scandinavica, 64,* 193-200.

Hagberg, B., Hagberg, G., & Olow, I. (1976). The changing panorama of cerebral palsy in Sweden—1954-1970): III. The importance of fetal deprivation supply. *Acta Pediatrica Scandinavica., 65,* 403-408.

Ingram, T. T. S. (1964). Cerebral palsy: Part I. *British Medical Journal, i.i.,* 1638-1640.

Ingram, T. T. S. (1965). Cerebral palsy: Part II. *British Medical Journal, i.i.,* 39-40

Prechtl, H. F. R. (1981). *Maturation and development: Biological and psychological perspectives.* London: Heinemann Medical Books.

Spinelli, D. N., Jansen, F. R., & Viana di Risco, G. (1980). Early experience effect on dendrite branching in normally reared kittens. *Experimental Neurology, 68,* 1-14.

Touwen, B. (1976). *Neurological development in infancy.* London: Heinemann Medical Books.

4

EARLY INTERVENTION FOR DISABLED CHILDREN IN THE CARIBBEAN

Marigold J. Thorburn

There are at least two serious misconceptions commonly held by human service professionals in health, education and social welfare services in developing countries, which have tended to obstruct the development of services to train and educate developmentally disabled children. These misconceptions are:

- handicapped children grow into dependent and non-productive adults, and therefore developing countries should not waste precious resources in providing training for them;
- training and education of handicapped children require highly specialized people working in a multidisciplinary team in a highly equipped center on a one-to-one basis, and are therefore very costly.

These two misconceptions lead to the conclusion that these services are not cost-benefical in developing countries. The first misconception contains a self-fulfilling prophecy which has already been disproved now that opportunities for development and training are being given to such children. Regarding the second, one of the major activities of the International Year of Disabled Persons (IYDP) was the dissemination of information about projects from all over the world, showing that it is possible to overcome this misconception. In fact, if developmentally disabled children in the developing world are to get any assistance at all, it is vital that we develop models that are low cost and can reach more children.

Over the past 10 years, several low cost projects providing early intervention have been started in the Caribbean. These projects operate in several different ways. The early stimulation projects in Jamaica and Curaçao provide intervention in the home by visitors. In Haiti the program is delivered in a clinic where parents bring their children to be advised and taught by the teaching staff of the special education school. Since 1982, this program has been extended with the help of UNICEF to an integrated day care program. Barbados also has a completely integrated early intervention program delivery in day care centers and residential homes for normal children. In these four countries 80-90% of the actual direct intervention work is done by para-professionals working under the supervision of a very small professional team.

In the Dominican Republic there is a variety of programs, one based in the maternity hospital which takes the child up to one and a half years, a second one involving home visiting as in Jamaica and Curaçao but using professional teachers, and a third one in a specialized center where the children come in daily for teaching. These projects use mainly professional staff, however, and so could not be classified as "low cost". This chapter will identify some of the constraints confronting these projects, how they are being tackled, some common needs identified, and future plans.

CONSTRAINTS OF OPERATING EARLY INTERVENTION PROJECTS IN THE CARIBBEAN

In developed countries, most people grow up in homes where welfare services, utilities and transportation are taken for granted. However, these basic essentials are frequently completely lacking in developing countries. Deprivation of stimulation in handicapped children is more often due to lack of knowledge and poverty than to deliberate neglect, but the result is the same—children are slow and regarded as dull or hopeless and thus function poorly. There is also now some research to suggest that some parents do not undergo the transition from simple bonding and loving their child to becoming the child's teacher (Bromwich, 1983).

Child rearing practices and lifestyles are also important. In the Caribbean, punishment is frequently used as a means of enforcing discipline and learning. Eventually the child becomes programmed to react only to threats and punishment. Attention-seeking behavior, non-compliance, and other behavior problems, such as self-stimulatory behavior may become evident. There is also the problem of the absent father, a situation which forces the mother to work to support the family. She may have very young children in the home at the same time with consequent reduction of the amount of time she can give to each one. Older children may have to stay away from school to take care of younger ones.

Families most in need of help with day care centers, health services, transportation and applicances, are the ones that have least access to them. These problems compound those of the disability and make them more difficult to solve and thus the family, like the disabled child, becomes handicapped.

Another feature of families afflicted by disability is the ignorance of cause and effect and the pervasive negative attitudes. The latter can be summarized as:

- misconceptions about etiology and superstitious beliefs relating to evil spirits, taboos, and resulting fear and guilt;
- the stigma of disability resulting in shame, concealment, and understimulation;
- the low expectations of the child resulting in deprivation of the normal opportunities available to the rest of the community;
- the lack of access to appropriate information, both for families themselves and for the basic human services that are available to such families.

The results of these negative conditions are that parents in poverty areas do not make efforts to help their children and do not advocate for their rights. They seem either to resign themselves to an unalterable situation and become apathetic about the child or direct their efforts to disposing of the child into the very sparse (and usually poorly run) institutions operated by government and charitable organizations. Miles (Chapter 7 in this volume) has written very lucidly of some of the cultural and religious practices in Asia influencing this situation.

Finally, services to meet childhood disability needs are few and often quite inappropriate for widely scattered rural populations. Most specialist services are centralized in capital towns. There are only three personnel training programs in the English speaking Caribbean and none in the French and Dutch speaking territories.

It is clear that alternative approaches are required. However, all the projects described here endorse the need for individual program planning and for regular and continuous contact with the family to maintain motivation and progress.

CARIBBEAN EARLY INTERVENTION PROGRAMS

JAMAICA

The aims of the Jamaican Early Stimulation Project which was started in 1975 are as follows:

- to mobilize parents of pre-school handicapped children to become the teachers of their own children in their own homes;
- to significantly improve the rate of development of such children; and
- to demonstrate that such a service can be provided at low cost by previously untrained community workers.

Jamaica has a population of just over two million people, one half in the urban area of Kingston and the other half in the rural areas. Racially the people are predominantly of black African origin, with a small percentage of Europeans, Chinese, East Indians and others. Until 1962, Jamaica was under British colonial rule.

The project is based on the Portage model of Wisconsin (Shearer & Shearer, 1972) which provides an early childhood education curriculum based on a precision teaching approach implemented in the home. Intervention is designed to meet the individual needs of the child, to capture the imagination of the mother and get her involved in the teaching process thus reinforcing the bonds of attachment between mother and child. The Portage model has been adapted to be used by a small team consisting of a doctor, public health nurse, teacher and sometimes a therapist, who train and supervise a larger team of community women, termed "child development aides".

These women had no previous formal training and had not received more than a 7th grade education. Special efforts were made to recruit parents of disabled children who have shown themselves to be skilled and motivated in handling their own children. More recently a training program for school leavers who reached grade 13 but did not have the academic pre-requisites for college or professional training has been developed. However maturity is a very important requirement.

The system used is as follows: First, the children needing help must be identified. They are usually recognized as being slow in development by mothers, family or friends. The mother will then consult a doctor, nurse or a clinic. Slowness in walking and other motor milestones are the most frequently noted early signs, for

Jamaicans have high expectations for motor development. Sometimes the child is identified as having a problem by a health worker on a routine visit to a clinic. This is particularly the case in the rural parishes where staff have become very sensitized to normal development and to early referral. The child is screened using the Denver Developmental Screening Test. If a significant delay in development is found, a full history, medical examination and developmental assessment is carried out. At this stage the program of intervention is designed by the professional team.

The intervention program is a combination of teaching, training and therapy carried out at home under the supervision of the child development aide. The most important aspect is that the mother gets fully involved in the program and carries out the teaching herself at home on a daily basis in between weekly visits by the aide. Finally, progress is reviewed and evaluated. This takes place at the office every 3-6 months. At this time the child may be referred to another specialist if desirable, or the program may be revised. In 1979, 36 children who had received an average of 35 months training on the project were reviewed. They learned on average 5.03 new skills per month, ranging from 1.5 to 10.1 new skills as compared with an expected rate of 6 to 8 skills per month for the normal child (Thorburn, 1981).

Between 1975 and the end of 1983 approximately 1,200 children under the age of 6 years with all types of disabilities were admitted to the project. Some of them have been in the program for only one or two months, while others have had four or five years of intervention.

The major causes of disability are prenatal and perinatal insults (approximately 45%). Postmeningitis brain damage and other infections account for about 11%, and genetic defects, particularly chromosomal abnormalities such as Down's Syndrome, account for approximately 20%. In approximately 20% of children the cause is not determined.

Training: Staff training was based on a task analysis of the expected role of the child development aide at the beginning of the project. Skills required for the task, as well as knowledge and background attitudes needed, were identified and a curriculum was drawn up including the teaching of such skills and knowledge. This resulted in an 8-week pre-service program broken down into the following topics:

- working with mothers and children;

- human relations;
- teaching techniques;
- normal child development;
- principles of behavior and its management;
- the characteristics of childhood disability;
- the Jamaican community, culture, social practices, and attitudes;
- services for handicapped children;
- making toys from junk material.

An evaluation of the project was conducted in 1983 for the Ministry of Social Security by a UNESCO consultant who strongly endorsed the project model and its efficiency in utilizing the community based approach. However, weaknesses existed mainly due to instability and insecurity of establishment as a government program and to inadequate financial support. As a result there has been irreparable attrition of staff, poor morale, and a fall in the quality of service.

A stronger professional team was recommended with the establishment of the child development aides as permanent workers. Unless this is done the future of the project looks bleak. At the time of writing the project serves children only in Kingston. A second project started in 1978 in an adjacent parish had to close due to lack of funds.

BARBADOS

The early stimulation program of the Barbadian Child Care Board, aimed at total integration, was launched in September, 1980 with sponsorship from UNICEF and consultation from the Caribbean Institute on Mental Retardation. The only one of its kind on the island, it began with training child care staff for government and private day care centers and children's homes; nurses, including public health nurses from the Ministry of Health, as well as parents were also trained. This was followed by a second training course in 1981. In all, a total of 69 persons have already received instruction.

The Child Care Board's program in its day care centers and residential homes involves the screening of children for disability using the Denver Screening Test, referral for medical assessment if needed, and the stimulation of those children detected to have problems. Catering for children three months to five years old, the program has led to better integration of the handicapped child in residential care and to the introduction of the principle of normalization and integration in day care facilities. The Board also works in collaboration with Ministry of Health personnel in polyclinics and its Developmental Center. Each of the Board's 15 day care centers accepts a maximum of six handicapped children. The current total is 77—less than the full capacity—and the board is committed to continuing the program.

CURAÇAO

Curaçao's Early Stimulation project was started in 1977 as part of the School Guidance Counseling Service, a government program. The project staff consisted of a coordinator and four home-teachers who worked closely with the baby clinic where the early detection was done. The Portage Guide, translated into Papamiento, was used as a model.

After seven years, the project is still part of the Guidance Service and in addition to the team, which has added a fifth home-teacher, a doctor checks all the children who may also be referred to a speech therapist. Weekly meetings are held with an orthopedic doctor who discusses not only the problems but their theoretical background with the workers. With 61 children now in the program, the team has good contact with related professionals such as those in kindergartens, school boards, day care centers, and other children's institutions.

HAITI

UNICEF is assisting in setting up a new program in Haiti in which people from all areas already working with children in their communities are being selected for training to become supervisors of day care facilities. The first training course lasts for three weeks, and from this, better selection processes are being developed. Three types of training are being offered:

- Groups to work with children 3-5 years old, both normal and handicapped. They are also taught how to detect disability.
- For children up to 2 years, or older ones not suited to the first type of training, trainees are taught individual stimulation using the Portage Guide. They also learn the DDST to detect disability.
- Treatment of both adults and children with disabilities

The third type of training has not come on stream as yet. The preschool (birth to 6 years old) is regarded as the priority in an area of immense need.

Training is held almost entirely in Port-au-Prince because of the expense and lack of facilities in rural areas. During the program's first year, 103 centers were opened in rural areas. Supervision is provided on an ongoing basis. The main priority of the program is prevention of disability. The major asset is that the centers are built on existing community resources, and they deal with all children, both disabled and non-disabled. The importance of having structured techniques to teach is also illustrated by the project. The program will serve 1.8% of Haiti's one million children in the 0-6 age group.

COMMON NEEDS, RESOURCES, AND APPROACHES

Research in early intervention is fraught with difficulties and complexities; there are so many variables at play (Gray & Wandersman, 1980) but the one general consensus is that it is beneficial. In addition to these difficulties well recognized in developed countries, developing countries have other constraints to face as outlined earlier.

Some of the common features of the Caribbean early intervention programs include poor economic and social resources, an ex-colonial background, use of the Portage Guide for Early Education, and dealing with all types of disabilities in the age group beginning from birth to 6. All except one country uses paraprofessionals.

During the past 2 years representatives of these projects have met twice to share ideas and approaches. One of the important issues that emerged was the technology that is used. The Portage Model is a very flexible, adaptable and practical one, and can be used in any setting. Although all projects were using unstandardized foreign tests, none felt very strongly that it was mandatory to standardize them, since the expense and time required would be difficult to justify. The service delivery model should be chosen according to the existing infrastructure in the country. Whichever is the most suitable and most feasible should be used to help the child develop in as integrated a setting as possible.

As for staffing, it was agreed that there was a need for at least two levels. The supervision and training should be provided by a "generalist professional" who could come from any human service background. A proposal for a regional training scheme for such a professional is now being prepared. The direct service staff can be paraprofessionals or "aides". Guidelines for the selection and training of these are being developed as well. The author believes that there is a third level required and that is the leadership person or project director. This person has to take the initiative and responsibility in developing and expanding the program.

Two other major areas of concern were parent motivation and participation and program evaluation. There is a need for more effective tools to assess parents' readiness to become their child's teacher and to monitor their adaptation and progress through the program. Better indices of the impact and effectiveness of intervention which are not just restricted to simple gains in any particular domain of development are very much needed in designing evaluations.

FUTURE DEVELOPMENT

Early intervention is still developing and experimenting with new strategies. It can be justified not only on the basis of the gains made by disabled children and the prevention of later adverse childhood complications, but also on the spin-off benefits that it provides in both teaching and childrearing techniques for normal children.

Finally, early intervention is feasible in almost any setting, although preference should be given to the most integrated situation possible. Integration is more difficult if the formal regular program has been in place for a long period of time. It therefore seems a good idea to try and develop these kinds of programs while the generic service programs are beginning, or shortly after.

There is another issue which is of concern to those who are aware of the constraints of developing new or expanded government programs. One of these is whether the existing primary health care worker or teacher can cope with an additional load for rehabilitation or early interevention. In Jamaica, experimental efforts in this direction have not been successful because there was no political or administrative policy to back up the project and the staff felt no compulsion to do the additional work. They therefore gave it up to other priorities. It does seem from the experience of community based rehabilitation that in order for primary health care workers to be able to carry out this type of work along with their other regular duties, they need to have a fairly small case load. They also need to spend a large proportion of their time in home visiting.

An advanatage of the home based type of program is that no special facilities are needed. All that is needed is an office with two or three rooms where children can be assessed, staff can meet, and toys and records can be kept. This office could be in any setting along with other services for children. However, we must also be aware of one of the serious disadvantages of community based programs. They do not have the visibility and high profile of institutional programs. This results in difficulties in fund raising from the usual charitable sources and no one notices when they "go under"—no one is seriously inconvenienced. Miles (Chapter 7 in this volume) presents a vivid and candid scenario of this situation in an analysis of community based rehabilitation.

New challenges continue to emerge. One is that we educate the public on the desirability of developing integrated community based programs. This is becoming more and more difficult. With the international shift to monetarism, the private sector is becoming more and more burdened and at the same time governments are containing and constricting the public sector. Our charitable sources are becoming drained before our governments are capable of taking over.

We now have the technology and the systems to effectively maximize the potential of the pre-school disabled child. The challenge is to find the resources, the arguments to justify their use, and the means to finance them.

References

Bromwich, R. (1983). *Parent behavior and progression: Manual and supplement.* Center for Research Development and Services, California State University, Northridge, California.

Gray, S.W. & Wandersman, L.P. (1980). The methodology of home based intervention studies: Problems and promising strategies. *Child Development, 51*, 993-1009.

Shearer, M. & Shearer D. (1972). The Portage Project: a model for early childhood education. *Exceptional Child, 36*, 210-217.

Thorburn, M. (1981). In Jamaica, community aides for disabled preschool children. *Assignment Children, 53/54*, 117-134.

5

A REALISTIC APPROACH TO THE PREPARATION OF PERSONNEL FOR REHABILITATION SERVICES IN DEVELOPING COUNTRIES

Marigold J. Thorburn & G. Allan Roeher[1]

INTRODUCTION

In developing countries, rehabilitation services are only just beginning and at present reach only 2% of disabled persons (WHO, 1981). This chapter, originally prepared in 1980, describes an approach for the preparation of all types and levels of personnel working in any type of human service which could be adapted to needs and resources in any part of the world. It has now been updated following the introduction of the notion of community based rehabilitation.

The approach is based on major concepts and principles developed in the western hemisphere and modified and tried in other parts of the world. It combines the manpower model developed in Canada in 1971 by the National Institute on Mental Retardation, the basic concepts and systems of competency-based education and task analysis, and the approach developed by the World Health Organization (WHO) known as Community Based Rehabilitation (CBR).

The Manpower Model was adopted by the International League of Societies for Persons with Mental Handicap (ILSPMH) in 1974, and the combination of the manpower model and competency-based education system (CBE) has been used to develop training programs for personnel in Barbados (Thorburn, 1982). Community based rehabilitation has been successfully tried and introduced into the island of St Lucia and had a successful trial in Jamaica where it has not yet been implemented.

---

[1]Deceased

PREREQUISITES TO DESIGNING TRAINING PROGRAMS

The question of training personnel in any field in countries where resources are limited requires investigation and planning. Before one can decide on the type of persons required and the kind of training that they will need, the scope and levels of services that already exist and that need to be provided must be identified. There are many complex issues which need to be taken into account and which must be dealt with if personnel to be trained are to be effective, efficient, and relevant to the needs of the country. So often people are sent away from developing to more developed countries to obtain long periods of training, and when they return they are helpless in dealing with the problems they encounter. They have been trained in traditional western models and are unable to adapt themselves to the problems and needs facing them in their own country. The result is that they become very dissatisfied. They may go elsewhere, they may return to the place of their training, perhaps enter private practice or, if they are lucky, enter a prestige disability center, a few of which have been established in developing countries.

Some of the issues which need to be considered include the following:

- the philosophy, goal, and policy for rehabilitation services;
- a knowledge of the needs in rehabilitation for solving the problems of disabled people in the countries concerned;
- the definition of the nature and scope of rehabilitation and its place within other human service systems;
- the need to use cost-beneficial approaches which will serve as wide a population as possible;
- the lack of specialized manpower and the need for development of a broader base of direct service workers with less training;
- the need for continuity of services both geographically and on a time continuum for all disability groups;
- the need for involvement of the people in the community and of disabled persons, in particular, in planning;
- the overall service delivery system; and
- the resources available.

PHILOSOPHY, GOALS AND POLICY

In the western world the philosophy of normalization and integration has been widely accepted. People with impairments have a right to the same services and place in society as does the normal person.

Bengt Nirje (1976) has said that the handicapped person has not just one handicap but three. The first is the impairment of function with which he is afflicted. The second is lack of opportunity and the restrictions placed on him by society who regard him or her as a burden and not a producer. This becomes a self-fulfilling prophecy. The third is the lack of self-esteem which eventually occurs when the disabled person begins to realize that he is regarded as a second-class citizen and useless to society.

As a result of society's negative attitudes, disabled people in the community have been segregated. In developing countries they may not have been institutionalized but they are frequently cut off from the mainstream of the community. We need to promote social integration through the development of services for disabled people in their communities, while at the same time helping them to develop their own potential. They should be participants in every aspect of normal life and have equal access to all services.

The goals for disabled people should be the same as those for normal persons, namely (briefly), to live a productive, happy, healthy, and integrated life in their own community.

NEEDS IN REHABILITATION

Here we are on slightly shaky ground in developing countries because we often do not have "needs data". We frequently have "head counts", as surveys may have been done, but these are not necessarily of much use for planning services. The WHO manual and the approach to community based rehabilitation has done much to clarify and simplify the differences in terminology which are being used and which help to understand and quantify the needs of disabled people with greater precision. Persons with exactly the same disability may have very different rehabilitation needs, as some may have rehabilitated themselves while others may need extensive retraining and adjustment of lifestyle. However, it can be said that most disabled people will need the following: early identification, diagnosis and medical treatment if at all possible; assessment of impairment of function; and an intervention program aimed at correction or remediation of the impairment.

Depending upon the severity and type of disability and the age of the person, the following services/programs may become necessary: early stimulation; parent training; counseling; behavior management;

appliances and aids; special education; therapy of various kinds; and possibly social support services, such as day care, welfare services, housing, or transportation. However, it is well recognized that the disabled person living in a rural area may not have access to many of these services. This is where community based rehabilitation services as delivered by community workers, may in fact be able to answer many of the needs stated above. The role of the CBR worker as advocated by WHO (1981) includes the identification of disabled people in the community, assessment of the disability, determination as to whether the disabled person needs training, planning a training program, identifying a trainer from the home, supervising them, evaluating progress and referring those disabled people requiring second level services. In addition, the local CBR worker has to be prepared to mobilize other community resources to facilitate social integration and access to regular health, educational and vocational activities.

It is not always necessary to undertake surveys in order to obtain information about rehabilitation needs. If records are kept with a view to future retrieval and use of such information, it may be possible to obtain the kind of data required by analysis of the clientele of clinics, schools, and other services which have been developed on an on going basis. However, if a program is definitively planned for a particular community, a survey of that community would be of great benefit, particularly if it is carried out by the people who are going to provide the service. Again the WHO manual provides information about carrying out a survey to generate "needs data".

DEFINITION OF REHABILITATION

A WHO Expert Committee recommended in 1981 the use of the following definitions (WHO, 1981):

> *Rehabilitation includes all measures aimed at reducing the impact of disabling and handicapping conditions, and at enabling the disabled and handicapped to achieve social integration. Rehabilitation aims not only at training disabled and handicapped persons to adapt to their environment, but also at intervention in their immediate environment and society as a whole in order to facilitate their social integration. The disabled and handicapped themselves, their families and communities in which they live should be involved in the planning and implementation of services relating to rehabilitation.*

As already mentioned, there is need for clarification in the terminology used relating to disability, handicap and impairment. Impairment and disability describe an abnormality of part of the body or bodily function which may affect important daily functions such as walking, moving, seeing, hearing, thinking, etc. It is only where there is a significant effect on activities of daily living that a person is said to be handicapped. It is therefore possible for a bilateral amputee, or a completely blind person not to be handicapped even though they have a severe disability.

COST-BENEFICIAL SERVICES TO REACH ALL

In the past, rehabilitatioin has been seen as a highly professionalized and specialized service with many vertical sub-specialties, including psychiatry, psychology, social work, at least three different species of therapists and many brands of special education. Clearly, this is an ideal completely out of reach for most developing countries which probably do not even provide professional training for more than one or two of those listed. CBR has fused all the above functions into a system which has several horizontal levels but in which the lowest or community level worker—termed the "local supervisor"—incorporates many of the skills but at a less complex level and geared towards solving problems faced in the community.

In most developing countries the few rehabilitation services available are tertiary level services provided by centralized institutions. In societies with limited resources, all must be used to the maximum. Cost-beneficial programs that reach larger numbers of people at the lowest cost possible must be developed. High quality rehabilitation only for the few who can afford it is, in our opinion, not acceptable as a major strategy in developing countries. Cost beneficial services are possible using the CBR approach.

BROADER BASED COMMUNITY SERVICES

As stated above, in more developed countries the main rehabilitation strategy has been the provision of highly specialized services with each professional taking a part or function of the body, such as the eye, the throat, hand or food, the brain, etc. Hopefully the person will be restored to a normal whole as a result of multiple assessments, prolonged case conferences, multiple referrals, extensive training programs, and expensive appliances! We accept that skilled professionals are needed, but they need to have a broader based supervision, with less day to day responsibilities for the provision of direct service needs of patients or clients. The bulk of the latter services can be undertaken by the CBR worker. This approach may also be relevant to more developed countries.

In 1971 an extensive study of manpower needs in mental retardation was carried out in Canada by the National Institute on Mental Retardation. This revealed that of all workers in services for the mentally retarded, 70% needed less than one or two years of training. Another 20 to 25 per cent needed three or more years (university level), and perhaps only 5% needed a masters degree or a Ph.D. for leadership positions. In addition it was recognized that not only was training important, but that personality and varying amounts of experience could balance more or less training. Figure 1 shows the manpower structure and its characteristics. This analysis has tremendous implication for personnel development in developing countries. It is probable that a similar structure and personnel needs are true, not only for Canada but for other countries and in other areas of service. The universality of the manpower concepts lies in its examination of the whole range of workers who are needed—from those who need very little training to those who require specialization. It is not an academic or professional model; rather it is a guide for ways by which a country can determine the kind of workers it needs based on the services required and the competencies available. From this approach it is possible for each country to decide on the amount and type of training needed for each of the four levels described. The more economically affluent nations have tended to stress higher academic requirements and therefore have a larger proportion of workers in Levels 2, 3, and 4, while developing countries tend to have fewer in the higher categories and stress short term training for basic direct care workers in Levels 1 and 2.

DETAILS OF LEVELS OF WORKER

Level 1 refers to the basic care workers, that is people who work under full supervision, sometimes known as "aides". They are also often volunteers. In the WHO approach they are the local supervisors who may be primary health care workers, teachers or people doing other jobs.

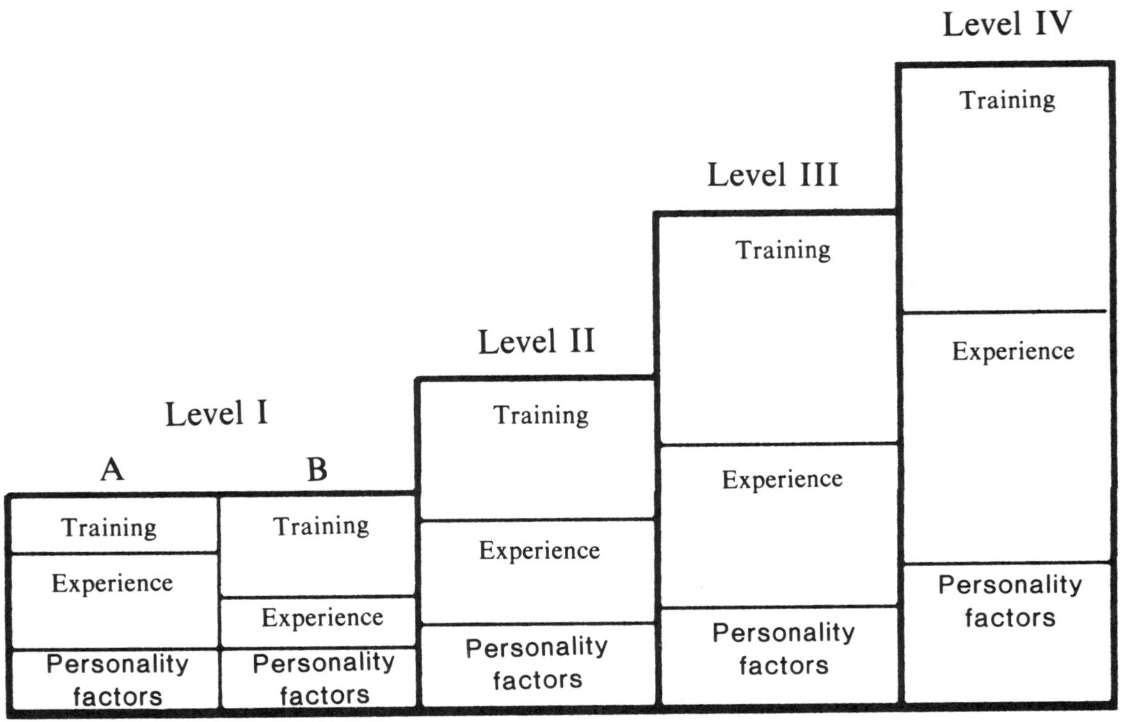

Figure 1. Career Ladder
Based on Canadian National Manpower Model,
National Institute on Mental Retardation (1971)

The level 2 worker needs to be able to give some supervision and is therefore a technician who obtains more theoretical instruction and practical learning than the level 1 worker. This could be obtained by one or two years of training or through on-the-job or in-service training over a period of time. This category would represent approximately 20% of the manpower force.

Level 3 consists mainly of technical staff, supervisory, and training personnel. Persons in this level could move up from Level 1 and 2 or receive formal pre-service training at an institution of higher learning such as basic university education with additional specialized training. This level would also include therapists who may have received training in a specialized college or school.

Level 4 includes those who are administrators, program planners, and other specialized professionals. People are in this level because they have had advanced training and/or extensisve experience. One of the requirements of a manpower model is the opportunity for workers to move from one level to another, ie. there must be professional advancement and upward mobility.

The ILSPMH has adopted this model and incorporated it into several training seminars and conferences and leaders from different countries have recognized the applicability of the model in their areas (Roeher, 1978). The Caribbean Institute on Mental Retardation and other Developmental Disabilities (CIMR) has applied the model with some success in helping to train personnel in different parts of the Caribbean, by means of short term modular training courses, (see Thorburn, 1982).

CONTINUITY OF SERVICES

Equitable distribution of services on a time and geographical continuum is probably the most difficult to achieve because it requires comprehensive rehabilitation planning which is not usually undertaken. This is necessary in order that disabled persons are not left out at certain times of their lives because they happen to live in a certain place or because they happen to have a certain type of disability. There must be a cooperative relationship between institutional and community services and between different sectors such as health, education, and labor. The objective should be that individuals get as much as possible what they most need to develop their potential and sustain their place in the community.

INVOLVEMENT OF THE COMMUNITY AND DISABLED PEOPLE

If the disabled are to be served in their own community, the resources and involvement of the community must be utilized. Although much lip service is often paid to efforts to get communities and community organizations involved in a meaningful and positive way to solve the problems of disabled people, such involvement may actually have the greatest benefit in changing negative attitudes. The exposure of people to positive action, and the resulting improvement through a participating relationship, could create positive reinforcement and thus more positive attitudes for all concerned. In addition many resources and developments which can be utilized may already exist at the grass roots level.

During the 1970s the Jamaica Association for Mentally Handicapped Children was able to extend the number of school places for mentally retarded children from 70 to nearly 900 throughout the island (Thorburn, 1979). Much of this expansion took place in rural areas in the regular school system. It happened without the provision of specialized teachers, psychologists or therapists. It happened because of the involvement and concern of community groups and the utilization of interested persons, such as teachers, public health nurses, and parents. Mobilization of all types of resources is clearly necessary.

Similarly, the participatory involvement of disabled persons themselves is essential. During the past four years the voice of disabled people has become stronger and more widely heard. Action groups may be few in developing countries but they are increasing in numbers and strength. If disabled persons are brought in as partners, and not just as the objects or recipients of services, the community will gain a potentially powerful resource.

In this context the guidelines for partnerships between developed and developing countries proposed by the ILSPMH are also very appropriate:

- assistance may be offered but not imposed;
- assistance must be genuine (not patronizing), have no hidden motives, and be intended only for the benefit of the handicapped and their families;
- decisions in the form of any voluntary society, the type and range of its services, its relationships with statutory authorities and others, must be made by the locals and not by outsiders;

- the pattern of services should be in accordance with local custom and culture, and its development should be at its own pace and its own way.
- indigenous staff, trained abroad if necessary, are preferable to imported staff;
- close contact must continue in a spirit of partnership with a two-way exchange of information, people and ideas.

The probability that rehabilitation strategies have already been devised by disabled people and their families cannot be ignored, and in this way disabled people themselves are invaluable resources (Werner, 1984).

OVERALL SERVICE DELIVERY SYSTEM

In this and in the consideration of training needs, we need to take another look at the concept of levels developed in the manpower model. This concept applies not only to personnel, but also to geographical distribution. These levels will therefore include:

- The simplest, cheapest, and those services reaching most people in the community. Community based rehabilitation clearly fits in at this level and would be provided by direct service workers such as primary health care workers, teachers and other volunteers in the community, including disabled people themselves.
- Middle level—more specialized, more complex, with more responsibility in training and supervision—would be at the parish or provincial level.
- Upper level, most specialized, most complex and regionally based.
- Leadership level—program planning, coordination, policy making, fiscal support—centrally placed.

This concept is familiar to health planners trying to develop a primary health care system on a tiered service delivery stystem. The CBR approach which originally only incorporated second level supervisors for the primary health care workers has recently been expanded to incorporate the higher level of organization as promoted here (Mendis, 1983).

EXISTING RESOURCES

Most countries, however poor, have some resources which can be utilized or developed to generate rehabilitation services. There may be a training program for social workers, public health nurses, or physiotherapists that could be strengthened for this purpose, or a primary health care system into which CBR could be incorporated. In St Lucia the primary health care service has been expanded to include rehabilitation. Training programs for nurses, school teachers and community health aides will be strengthened by the addition of appropriate knowledge and skills. In Haiti (see Chapter 4 in this volume) community day care providers are being trained to provide care and education for disabled as well as normal children. In the Philippines (Periquet, 1984) community volunteers have been trained as local supervisors and work without pay.

SELECTION AND TRAINING OF PERSONNEL

Taking into account the issues and constraints discussed above, it is now possible to look at the manpower needs and the required training. Steps to the design of training programs will include the following:

A precise definition of the service to be provided: The tasks that will be performed need to be analyzed and the personnel and their resources and skills defined. This is essentially a task analysis of jobs to be done and the skills that will be needed to carry out those tasks.

Examination of the available resources: The competencies of the persons available to carry out the tasks will also need to be defined. What will these people need to learn to be able to carry out the tasks? Bearing in mind the manpower model, the basic characteristics of personality will affect the selection of suitable candidates, and the provision of varying levels of modules of training can lead to the achievement of the desired competencies. Is the service to be started completely from scratch or will personnel who are to carry out the tasks already be in a service? This is particularly relevant in developing countries where personnel are in short supply and rehabilitation services are only just beginning. To try to superimpose a rehabilitation model on service systems which are scanty is unrealistic. The staff may not be able to undertake the additional tasks.

The total system must be examined: This will include four components in addition to the question of personnel already mentioned: a) The place or site where the service is to be provided; b) the program that will be implemented; c) the clientele to be served, their problems, age, geographical distribution; and d) the system in which the service operates, its links with other services, points of entry and discharge, etc.

Ideally it would be better to build on the skills of personnel in existing systems. However, for the reasons given above, these systems are sometimes so rigid or the staff already so overworked, that it is impossible to incorporate a totally new set of tasks. In this instance a separate model could be built which would be adapted and eventually incorporated into the regular system if it is found to be effective. An example of this is the Early Stimulation Project in Jamaica (see Chapter 4). Here it proved impossible to develop the project within the existing services of either Health or Education. It was therefore piloted by the Jamaica Council for the Handicapped under the Ministry of Social Security. Since that time, efforts have been made to replicate the service in other situations using existing health personnel. This has not been successful so far and the Ministry of Health has reinstated the integration of the program into its community health service. Community based rehabilitation has also been attempted in a parish where the number of health staff available is relatively high in proportion to the members of the community being served. It proved to be entirely feasible.

Design of Training: Skills and knowledge to be learned can now be listed, analyzed and sequenced in order of priority. Each skill or area of knowledge can be taught in modules. The depth of skill or number of skills required can be defined for each level of staff. It would then be possible to develop a core training program which all levels of staff would need, as well as other more specialized or in-depth modules for other or higher levels of staff, or perhaps more extensive time may be devoted to practical skills required by lower level direct service workers (Thorburn, 1982).

When new staff are being trained for a totally new service, it has been found beneficial for the supervisory staff themselves to help to design and conduct training for the field staff. This can be done through task analysis and by having the staff participate in the actual training and teaching of the skills to lower level staff.

It will be clear that this approach requires detailed planning, a thorough knowledge of the tasks to be performed, and time to do it. Time spent in planning is often neglected and regarded as unnecessary. Attention to detail, however, is important and pays off in the long run as it is often found that the planned time frame set for training can sometimes be shortened, because skills are more logically taught and are therefore learned more easily.

Finally, it has been found by many people working in the rehabilitation field in the broadest sense (Mittler, 1979) that the behavioral approach and the teaching of the principles and practical applications of behavior modification is a very productive area of training. This is probably because the behavioral approach is essentially a problem-solving one and once personnel can be taught problem-solving skills, they can tackle almost any problem. In fact, the manpower model is based on the ability of various levels of staff to solve the problems of those whom they supervise. In theory therefore, it should be possible to train almost anyone, almost anywhere, to do almost anything!

IMPLEMENTATION OF TRAINING PROGRAMS

Many strategies for implementing training programs are available (Lugo, 1978, Roeher, 1979, Mittler, 1979). A country or local area can select or develop the one that best suits its needs and resources. For each area, persons who know well the local services, customs, and culture need to work closely with those with the specialized skills to be taught and the planner who knows and can put into effect the principles and practical strategies of training. Countries with limited resources in the two later areas can draw on a number of international resources to assist them. In many countries, Peace Corps Volunteers can provide technical skills to assist local leaders with planning. In the western hemisphere, the Partners of the Americas Program has provided, in a unique way and on a country to country basis, skilled input in planning and training (Thorburn, 1977). Similar relationships are being developed through the ILSPMH between African and Asiatic and European countries.

In order to mobilize these resources and monitor programs, a technical entity may sometimes be required. The Caribbean Institute on Mental Retardation (CIMR) is an example of such an entity. The institute has been successful in mobilizing international support for, and technical cooperation between 25 or so small countries in the Caribbean basin. In the past, many services in developing countries have been designed by foreign experts which, when implemented were found not to be realistic or to meet the needs of the country because of the inadequacy of local resources. Because one model suited one country it may not necessarily be successful when replicated in another. Failure to evaluate or take into account local constraints or needs may account for this. Each country needs to develop its own model using general principles. A regional resource center in collaboration with a national resource center or institute, whose main functions are to provide information, training, access to technical expertise and consultations could be very helpful in facilitating program development as described here (CIMR Quadrennial and Biannual Reports, 1980, 1982, 1984)[2]

CONCLUSION

Ideally, the design and implementation of training programs are carried out as suggested here in the complete knowledge of the context of the existing infrastructure and with the full participation of all sectors involved. One wonders how often this is done in real life and if so, whether it is evaluated. As stated in the introduction, most developing countries are only just beginning to move into rehabilitation. This very evolutionary step may indicate a concern for the quality of life which might be a valid indicator of a country's level of development.

The purpose of this chapter therefore is to indicate how that step might be taken in a planned and rational fashion so that a well integrated system develops which does not exhibit the usual overlaps and gaps characteristic of rehabiliation services in many countries. It must be admitted that the authors are not aware of any country in which this ideal situation exists!

References

Lugo, D.E. (1978). *A new alternative for the training of personnel for handicapped children.* Paper presented at the First World Congress on Special Education, Stirling Scotland.

---

[2]These reports are obtainable from the CIMR, 6 Courtney Drive, Kingston 10, Jamaica.

Mendis, P. (1983). *Community based rehabilitation.* Paper presented at the Conference of the Caribbean Association of Rehabilitation Therapists, Kingston, Jamaica.

Mittler, P. (1979). *Strategies for manpower development in the 1980s.* Paper presented at the Fifth International Congress of the International Association for the Scientific Study of Mental Deficiency (IASSMD), Jerusalem, Israel.

National Institute on Mental Retardation, Canada (1971). *A National mental retardation manpower model.* Toronto: NIMR.

Nirje, B. (1976). *The normalization principle: Patterns which are changing.* Paper given at a meeting sponsored by the President's Committee on Mental Retardation and the International League of Societies for Persons with Mental Handicap (ILSPMH), Fairlie, Virginia, U.S.A.

Periquet, A. (1984). *Community based rehabilitation services: The experience of Bacolod, Philippines and the Asia-Pacific Region.* (Monograph #26). New York: World Rehabilitation Fund.

Roeher, G. A. (1978). *Choices in the preparation of personnel in mental retardation and developmental disabilities—a planned approach to meeting international needs.* Paper presented at the Fifth Congress of the International League of Societies for Person with Mental Handicap, Vienna, Austria.

Roeher, G. A. (1979). *A balanced approach to personnel preparation and utilization in developed and developing countries.* Paper given at the Fifth Congress of the International Association for the Scientific Study of Mental Deficiency, Jerusalem, Israel.

Thorburn, M. J. (1977). *Small is beautiful.* A contribution to a plenary panel at the Annual General Meeting of the Partners of the Americas, Santo Domingo, Dominican Republic.

Thorburn, M. J. (1978). *Simplified special education— a working model for the Caribbean.* Paper given at the UNESCO Expert Meeting on Special Education, Paris, France.

Thorburn, M. J. (1979). *Early stimulation for handicapped children using community workers.* Paper given at the Fifth Congress of the International Association for Scientific Study of Mental Deficiency, Jerusalem, Israel.

Thorburn, M. J. (1982). *Training of child care staff for integrated programs for pre-school handicapped children.* Paper presented at the Sixth Congress of the International Association for the Scientific Study of Mental Deficiency, Toronto, Canada.

Werner, D. (1984). *Project Projimo: An article in aids to living.* London: AHRTAG.

WHO (1981). *Training the disabled in the community: A manual (2nd. Ed.).* Geneva: World Health Organization.

6

SERVICE DELIVERY SYSTEMS AND COMMUNICATION DISORDERS IN DEVELOPING AFRICAN COUNTRIES

Elizabeth T. I. Akpati

INTRODUCTION

One of the increasingly poignant common denominators among developing African countries is the plight of those with varying forms of handicapping conditions. Rapid increases in the number of handicapped persons in these countries, stem largely from nutritional deprivation and inadequate health care delivery systems which do not effectively provide for early detection, prevention of diseases, and the rehabilitation of individuals who are disabled.

A handicapping condition is one that renders the individual incompetent in mental, communicative, physical, or socio-emotional abilities to such an extent that the individual is deviant from the homogenous group or the so-called *normal* population, and requires a program of special education, rehabilitation or other social services in order to develop to the fullest potential.

In many advanced countries, it is generally accepted by the public that a certain minimum standard of living must be available to all members of a community, and if poverty prevents its attainment by an individual, the local, state, or federal government is expected to provide it. The rehabilitation of handicapped children, for example, is not left totally to parents or family members. The government assumes a great deal of responsibility in the care, education or rehabilitation of the handicapped. In sub-Saharan African countries, there is little understanding of the many disadvantages associated with the life circumstances of the disabled. Although authorities in government make pronouncements that opportunities for personal growth and advancement should be open to all, handicapped persons are at a great disadvantage when it comes to a fair distribution of financial resources to meet their needs. It is difficult for African governments to justify allocating huge financial resources for the establishment of special programs for the disabled population when the majority of the able-bodied population are overwhelmed by a multitude of obstacles in their way to social advancement.

The general relationship between poverty and disease is reflected in the health indices of all developing countries. People suffer ill-health because they are poor and they are rendered even poorer because they are sick, and so the vicious cycle continues to depress living standards. Poor sanitation and malnutrition escalate the most commonplace illness or injury into a serious threat to life. Preventable communicable diseases such as malaria, small-pox, tuberculosis, cholera, measles, meningitis, etc. form the greater part of the medical problem in Africa because of inadequate recognition of the relationship between disease and the physical environment. Although many of the so-called tropical diseases are thought to be confined to the tropics, they were widespread in the temperate zones of the world where they caused devastation until drastic improvements were made in the physical environment (Davey, 1958). England and many parts of Europe were devastated by epidemics of malaria, yellow fever, leprosy, tuberculosis, thyphus, and relapsing fever in the late 1930s until efficient control methods became available. Thus, sickness and death from these etiologies declined when the living conditions of the working population improved through better housing, better sewage disposal, pure water supplies, and better nutrition.

Despite the fact that health has come to occupy a very high place on the priority list of many African governments, the level of infrastructure for basic health services has remained low as a result of several factors. The first is the inheritance of curative medicine from the colonial era. The preservation of the health of the European minority was of key concern to the colonial administration because the coastal areas where the administrative centers were located posed a very serious health hazard to the Europeans due to the prevalence of malaria and other tropical diseases (Gish, 1980). This orientation to curative medicine has led to the persistence of major communicable diseases which account for a high incidence of disabilities and mortality. The 1977 Medical Survey of Nigeria estimated that half the annual deaths in Nigeria occur among children between one and five years of age with a mortality rate of 180 per 1000 live births. Although diseases such as small pox have been eradicated or their incidence greatly diminished by vaccination, measles, cerebrospinal meningitis, and malaria are still widespread and account for a high mortality rate.

Another legacy left by the old colonial administration and one that has had a deleterious effect on the overall health care delivery in many African countries is the gross maldistribution of health facilities and health personnel. As Marfo (Chapter 1 in this volume) points out, there is a marked disparity in the provision of health services in urban and rural areas. First and foremost, the colonial administration was concerned with the acquisition of choice lands for the production of export crops. Secondly, it was concerned with the preservation of the health of the European minority and since the administrative centers were based in urban areas, port cities, and mining towns, the principal health facilities were strategically clustered in these administrative centers to serve the needs of the European community

This bias toward urban-based health facilities, coupled with poor transportation, led to the inaccessibility of these health services to rural areas where the vast majority of the population reside. In Nigeria, it is estimated that western medicine reaches only about 25% of the population (Nelson, 1982). The inbalance between curative and preventive medicine, and between health care delivery in urban and rural areas still persists in ways very reminiscent of the colonial period.

SERVICE DELIVERY AND THE STATE OF THE ECONOMY

The economic situation in which many African countries have found themselves has a bearing on the expenditure for health and human services. Much of the economy of African countries depended on agricultural resources. However, in the last decade, the rural oriented economy and subsistence farming have given way to an urbanized economic structure. In 1970, domestic revenues in Liberia amounted to $66.5 million and the total national expenditures for health was $4.8 million or 7.4% of the total national budget (U.S. Department of Health Education & Welfare, 1973). In the 1973-74 fiscal year, the total national budget of Ghana was 759.3 million cedis of which only 7.2 million cedis were allocated to health (U.S. Department of Health Education & Welfare, 1974). Although specific figures relative to Nigeria's expenditure for health are not available, inferences can be made that they are not much greater than those of Ghana and Liberia. Fund allocations are inadequate in view of the magnitude of health problems in these countries. The total funds allocated to health on the one hand and their distribution on the other have serious implications for the development of significant public health programs. Nigeria used to be mostly agrarian; however, agriculture which is the mainstay of the population has given way to urban industrialization and declined to the point where the country now cannot produce enough food for domestic consumption and has become a major food importer. The rapid emergence of oil in the mid-1970s placed Nigeria in very favorable economic circumstances. Nigeria's Third National Development Plan (1975-1980) embarked on a national development of major proportions. Included in this plan was a strong commitment to improve the standard of living of its people and to make education available to all, including the handicapped.

Unfortunately, the volatile nature of the international oil market brought about decreased demand for oil and subsequent decrease in production. Against this background of global depression, particularly in the economies of industrialized nations, financial resources necessary for implementing major long-term objectives became scarce. Nigeria and many African countries have been forced to engage in massive borrowing from overseas markets and from multilateral organizations such as the World Bank. Faced with pressing national priorities, health and human services for the disabled remain at the lowest end of national development plans and suffer glaring serious disproportions in the allocation of financial resources. With little education, the disabled have no place in this new fabric of society.

ILLITERACY

Of the factors concerned in establishing adequate health services, ignorance is perhaps the most common and the most difficult to eradicate. Education has not been fully employed for the promotion of positive health behaviors among all segments of the population through heightened public awareness and increased availability of information and resources. Although education is a high priority in the development plans of many African nations, huge populations remain functionally illiterate in an era when the continent is going through urban development and blue collar jobs.

The electronic media (radio and television) have not been effectively utilized as a weapon against mass illiteracy, ignorance, and poverty, and have not made contributions toward raising the level of information among those who cannot read printed words. Rather, the electronic media have been used as a political showpiece to demonstrate the progressive nature of leaders and as a device for the importation of foreign entertainment. There is a lack of understanding of the nature and special characteristics of the electronic media as a means of communication and education under conditions entirely different from those in which they have functioned in more advanced countries.

With the alarming rate of illiteracy in African countries and with relatively few people who speak the official languages (English, French or Portuguese), the electronic media could contribute significantly to the solutions of the problem of chronic shortage of well-trained teachers and as a tool for social education and community development.

COMMUNICATION DISORDERS

The present day concept of rehabilitation encompasses the provision of comprehensive services to enable those with handicapping conditions to achieve maximum personal, social, and economic independence so that they can be absorbed within the mainstream of society. Of the various types of handicapped persons, those with communication disorders are among the most neglected. Treatment of communication disorders, as an aspect of health care, is still very new in many African countries, and data on the subject are very limited. At the present time, there seems to be little interest by those in government and by physicians and psychologists to embark on comprehensive programs in the areas of research, training, or clinical services for those with speech, language, and hearing disorders.

The professions of speech pathology and audiology exist in only a few institutions of higher learning in Nigeria and Ghana although the first schools for the deaf have been in existence in Lagos and Accra since 1957, as a result of the initiative of philanthropic organizations and missionaries who somehow saw the need to provide these services. But such early institutions were no more than sanctuaries which isolated the deaf and left them unprepared for living in society. Without the availability of speech pathology and audiology services, those with communication disorders resulting from primary etiologies are left to physicians who refer these cases to otolaryngologists who in turn are ill-equipped and not adequately trained to take on the added burden of providing clinical management. Emphasis thus far has been on treating the underlying causes of communication disorders.

Late identification of a hearing loss among children is a concern of major proportions in African countries. The first five years are the most formative in a child's development and are the critical years for speech and language learning. When a hearing loss is not identified early, the chances of rehabilitation are decreased. The result is that such children become unproductive citizens and a major source of economic strain on the meager financial resources of their families. Deafness has been considered mainly as a medical problem and thus, the focus of otolaryngology has been one of a health preserving profession and there has been less concern to a large degree with the restoration of function. The disorder has the potential for considerable risk to life and bodily harm and severe socio-economic repercussions. There needs to be concern in treating not only the underlying etiologies but also the associated communication disorders.

A review of the literature shows that there has been a long history of interest in African countries in providing rehabilitation services for the orthopedically handicapped, the deaf, and the blind, with the help of both government and charitable organizations. However, services for those with communication disorders exist on a minimal scale. Little attention has been given to speech, language, and less severe forms of hearing impairments. In the area of hearing, the development of education, training and vocational programs has been geared mainly to the needs of the profoundly deaf; programs for individuals who are partially deaf are virtually nonexistent. However, the partially deaf constitute a large population of handicapped persons for whom services need to be provided. There is often a lack of awareness of the limitations that communication disorders impose upon the proper development and social adjustment of the individual.

Many of us have varying concepts of communication, depending on our educational or professional orientation. Regardless of our definitions of communication (either as a means by which we receive or send messages, or as a medium by which we achieve psycho-social interaction), we must all admit that the inability to engage in it is a social isolation and a world of limited experience. As a social function, communication makes significant contributions to intellectual functioning and is an occupational necessity which is essential to effective day to day living.

What accounts for the fact that African countries are still at the baseline of dealing with the problem of communication disorders and do not fully appreciate the adverse effects of congenital or acquired speech, language or hearing disorders? Efforts to make advancements in agricultural and industrial developments have contributed to the apparent oversight in meeting the needs of individuals with communication disorders. Although it has been well-documented that childhood diseases which may arise as early as the first week of fetal life can cause hearing, language, or speech defects, still a large majority of these cases do not receive early evaluation or treatment. The medical profession has done very little in providing rehabilitation services for those with communication disorders beyond its responsibility of simply providing narrowly conceived medical or surgical treatment.

PREVALENCE OF COMMUNICATION DISORDERS

No one is sure of the extent of speech, language, and hearing disorders among children and adults in Africa or the number of persons who receive some form of remedial or other social services. The various types of communication disorders on the continent are similar to those found anywhere in the world, but their prevalence may vary from one African country to another and from those found in industrialized countries. There is a tendency for people not to seek medical help unless the hearing impairment is of sudden onset or is accompanied by severe or unusual symptoms such as vertigo or tinnitus (Fajemisin, 1980). Even though estimates of hearing disorders are not exactly known, there is ample evidence in the literature that indicates that cerebrospinal meningitis, a major killer, is a leading cause of deafness in most African countries lying between the Sahara desert to the north and the equatorial forest to the south (WHO, 1969). A variety of other diseases such as small-pox, measles, mumps, and influenza are widespread in West and Central Africa and are major causes of deafness.

ATTITUDES TOWARD THE SPEECH AND HEARING IMPAIRED

Individuals with communication disorders do not enjoy the same consideration in terms of rehabilitation services as those with visible handicaps such as the blind or the orthopedically-impaired. The amputee, the quadriplegic, or the blind person with a cane gets immediate attention and sympathy because his/her handicap is conspicuous and so his/her needs are, in some measure, appreciated. But those who are deaf or lacking in communication ability appear outwardly normal until they attempt to speak. They arouse a negative response in the form of patronization and ridicule.

Social degradation attends speech and hearing defects in African countries. The hard-of-hearing are shouted at and there are jokes about them as having 'hard-ears.' Stutterers are often ridiculed and a child with a less severe form of mental retardation may be regarded as 'lame-of-mind'. All forms of malocclusions abound, and the resultant articulation problems which could be alleviated through surgical or prosthetic management, attract attention and ridicule.

Of the handicapped population, the group that is subjected to the worst form of social degradation is the so-called 'deaf and dumb' or 'deaf-mute.' These are persons who are congenitally deaf or who, at a very early age, acquired deafness before the critical period of language learning. Unfortunately, this nomenclature is sometimes used by professionals who are knowledgeable about communication disorders in order to make themselves understood by the general public. Many of these children who are classified as 'deaf and dumb' have never experienced any input via the sensory channel of hearing and, thus, they are unable to speak or understand audible speech. The term designates two disabilities: the first is a primary problem of sensory loss of hearing and the second is a secondary problem of the inability to use speech. The child is unable to speak because of deafness and not because he is dumb or stupid. Until deafness, speech and language are closely related to one another, there will remain a lack of awareness that the ear serves as the channel through which we learn to talk, and that a serious hearing defect will result in defective speech and delayed language.

The negative association of the word 'dumb' with deafness may have severe socio-economic repercussions and some far-reaching implications for other handicapping conditions. For example, the laryngectomized person or the aphasic stroke patient may be classified as 'deaf and dumb' simply on the basis of the individual's inability to communicate. Many children who are so classified may not really be totally deprived of all sensory stimuli but have some useful residual hearing. For children in this category, speech and language development is fundamentally different from that of children who are congenitally deaf. And thus, a differential diagnosis is very important to distinguish those who are actually deaf from those who are not, so that appropriate therapeutic management and social services could be provided.

The research output has not been proportionate to the magnitude of the clinical and psychosocial problems related to these communication disorders. The literature is replete with findings which show that sensory deprivation of any particular modality may precipitate catastrophic reactions in the individual. Deafness and severe speech defects affect the totality of the entire being. The individual may function below his potentialities.

RECOMMENDATIONS AND RESEARCH NEEDS

An attempt has been made in this chapter to shed some light on the dynamics operating in the delivery of health services for the disabled in African countries and how they impact on service delivery in relation to communication disorders. The foregoing observations are by no means exhaustive but serve to illustrate the need for the establishment of speech and hearing services in the developing regions of the continent. On that basis, the following recommendations for development are offered:

1. Demographic data are problematic in many African countries. Given the limited fragments of information and the scarcity of reliable scientific data on the prevalence of handicapping conditions including communication disorders, national surveys to quantify the types and distribution of these disorders require priority attention as an essential element in providing rehabilitation services.

2. There needs to be awareness by authorities in the government that a national policy which tends to keep the individual healthy and at work raises the productivity of the community and its wealth. To this end, there has to be a shift in focus from curative to preventive medicine. The strong emphasis on curative health services in a continent where communicable diseases are widespread must be closely scrutinized if there is to be a reasonable improvement in the overall health of the African people. Investing in preventive health services will minimize the incidence of childhood diseases. There is no doubt about the potential trade-off between the high cost of curative health services that benefit a minority of urban populations and preventive health services that could reach the majority of the people, especially those in the rural areas. Ministries of health should be involved in developing and organizing peripheral networks of speech and hearing services in the form of mobile units to reach the majority of populations which are geographically truncated from the major urban-based health services and trading institutions.

3. Perhaps the greatest need is improved public health education and applied nutrition. Mental retardation and structural abnormalities which preclude the development of normal speech and language may be traceable to malnutrition going back to the prenatal period. Malnutrition should always be blamed on poverty, although ignorance and superstition are major factors in malnutrition in some communities. Rural communities should be given instruction in health education to promote good nutritional habits.

4. Medical practitioners and the public are not fully aware of the necessity for early diagnosis of speech and hearing disorders. There is a tendency for most parents to wait till the speech or hearing handicapped child is two years old or of school-going age before seeking medical help, in the hopes that the child will speak with maturation. This lack of awareness emphasizes the need for disseminating pertinent information among the community and practicing physicians on the implications of speech and hearing disorders.

5. A speech or hearing handicap has many facets and so a collaborative effort is important in finding solutions to the problem. Unless disciplines such as otolaryngology or neurology seek cooperation from allied professions, they would continue on their present course as independent disciplines, implementing their own isolated research; consequently, solutions would take a longer time to reach.

6. There is the need for the development of comprehensive training and clinical speech and hearing services. The responsibility of coordinating and running the clinical programs should rest on trained and qualified professionals in the field of communication disorders rather than on medical practitioners who do not have the adequate knowledge of or training in Speech Pathology and Audiology. The services these physicians provide are only peripheral to their primary health care responsibilities.

7. Finally, cross-cultural collaborative research is needed to enhance the pool of information on the disease processes which produce various forms of communication disorders among Africans.

References

Davey, T. H. (1958). *Disease and population pressure in the tropics*. Ibadan: Ibadan University Press.

Fajemisin, B. (1980). Comment on O. L. Taylor's "Communication disorders in blacks." In B. E. Williams & O. L. Taylor (Eds.), *Working papers: International Conference on Black Communication, August, 1979*. New York: Rockefeller Foundation.

Gish, O. (1980). Review of cross-national study of health system. In R. Ingram & A. E. Thomas (Eds.), *Topics and Utopias in health*. The Hague: Mouton Press.

Nelson, H. (1982). (Ed.), *Nigeria: A country study*. Washington, D. C.: American University Foreign Area Studies Department.

U.S. Department of Health, Education, and Welfare (1973). *Syncrisis: The dynamics of health: An analytic series on the interactions of health and socio-economic development, VII: Liberia*. Washington, D. C.: HEW Office of International Health.

U.S. Department of Health, Education, and Welfare (1974). *Syncrisis: The dynamics of health: An analytic series on the interactions of health and socio-economic development, X: Ghana*. Washington, D. C.: HEW Office of International Health.

WHO (1969). Cerebrospinal meningitis in Africa. *WHO Chronicle, 23*(2), 54-64.

7

MISPLANNING FOR DISABILITIES IN ASIA

M. Miles

INTRODUCTION

Pakistan and its immediate neighbors, India, China, Afghanistan and Iran, make up a sizeable proportion of Asia both in area and in their combined population of 2 billion. Rehabilitation work suffered during the internal problems in Iran and will presumably take some years to pick up again. The joint initiative to set up in Teheran an International Center for the Study of Rehabilitation in Developing Countries unfortunately never reached a useful functioning level. (It is to be hoped that the experience gained will be deployed in another country with better results.) In Afghanistan the need for rehabilitation of disabled persons barely gains official recognition (spokesmen at international gatherings have been known to state that there is little disability among Afghans since the Revolution has solved all the problems of the people). A small effort is being made in Kabul for the rehabilitation of blind and physically disabled persons.

In China there have been some experimental classes for mentally retarded children, some special schools for mixed disabilities, the treatment of hearing loss with acupuncture, and nation-wide efforts to prevent disabilities by basic hygiene and improved midwifery. It seems unlikely that the Chinese Government will be seduced into setting up expensive prestige projects for the handicapped. On the contrary, the WHO Community Rehabilitation schemes might find very fruitful ground in the existing extensive primary health care system. A similar conclusion was reached by Dixon (1981) after a detailed study in China.

Rehabilitation facilities in India are 20 or 30 years ahead of developments in Pakistan, but mostly in a direction that would seem regressive to Western rehabilitation advisors. The International Year of Disabled Persons (IYDP) saw a new crop of grandiose schemes for immense residential projects, even a whole 'disabled village'. India is so large that there is little effective central co-ordination. The Federal Government tried to promote integration of handicapped children into regular schools by the offer of large-scale aid to set up such schools. There were hardly any takers over a 5-year period. However, there are sufficient indigenous resources of experience, equipment and specialist staff, and therefore any serious rehabilitation policy should be able to yield good results.

This chapter is based on a paper written after three years of working with handicapped children in the North West Frontier Province of Pakistan, running special schools, advising the Government on the most appropriate strategies for developing facilities for handicapped persons, and attending professional conferences on the subject. The immediate spurs were: a) a month-long trip through India visiting rehabilitation centers and attending a major Congress and a workshop on epidemiology, financed by the Rosemary Dybwad International Award; b) an evaluation exercise on the new WHO Community Rehabilitation manuals; c) discussions on development with UN advisers in other fields; and d) the discovery that five Western rehabilitation advisers visiting Pakistan earlier had given mutually contradictory advice.

During the past three years which included the International Year of Children (IYC) and the International Year of Disabled Persons (IYDP), there has been much talk about handicaps in Pakistan, and I have contributed my share of comment and advice to the Government, along similar lines to that made by the WHO, UNICEF, Rehabilitation International and other bodies with world-wide experience.

There are three broad trends in Pakistan at present in the development of special education and rehabilitation. There is a move to improve and expand existing facilities for special education. Plans are being implemented to build huge 'Disability Complexes'. The WHO Community Rehabilitation scheme is appearing on the horizon. Pakistan is a sufficiently large nation for there to be room for several different initiatives in developing facilities for handicapped persons. Nevertheless, the lack of coordination between the three trends is damaging to all, and they will inevitably be in competition for official backing and resources. It is therefore worth while examining these trends to see why they are taking place, and what is their likely outcome.

The following discussion is relevant to much of Asia, and also to some other parts of the less developed world. No attempt has been made to follow WHO's use of the terms impairment, disability, and handicap. In Pakistan we are at the stage of terminology where the 1981 National Census included a question listing disabilities thus: 1) Blind; 2) Deaf and Dumb; 3) Crippled; 4) Mad (Urdu—*Pagal*); 5) Half Mad (Urdu—*Nim Pagal*, to denote mental handicap); 6) other.

The Government's intention to improve existing facilities has been laudable, but by and large, implemented in a naive fashion so that handicapped adults and children themselves have seen very little benefit from it. The exercise has been run 'from the top downwards' with a strong smell of money sloshing about, in the worst tradition of development aid. There has been no coordination between the Ministry of Education, the Ministry of Health and Social Welfare and the National Council for Social Welfare, each of which runs its own show and makes its own plans with a spirit of rivalry rather than co-operation. This lack of coodination resulted, for example, in the National Council for Social Welfare's not being invited to send a representative to the National IYDP Committee, and in the setting up of no less than three independent prosthetics workshops in one year in one provincial capital, amidst bitter competition for trained staff, while nothing had been planned for the rest of the Province. Courses in speech therapy were provided for teachers of the deaf, but apparently nobody in the Ministry concerned realized that speech therapy also plays a major part in rehabilitation of the mentally retarded. A survey of physically disabled children in regular schools got lost in the backwash of petty bureaucracy and inter-departmental jealousies.

PRESTIGE DISABILITY COMPLEXES

Nobody seems to know just how many grandiose schemes are afoot for Disability Complexes. The Education Ministry and the Ministry of Health and Social Welfare appear to be running parallel schemes in mutual ignorance. The Islamabad Capital Development Authority may have its own scheme, or it may turn out to be part of a Ministry scheme. One Complex will probably be part of a gargantuan National Hospital, and another complex is half-way to completion in Baluchistan. All these complexes have been planned and undertaken either in ignorance or in flat contradiction of the advice given by international agencies in the rehabilitation field. It is of interest, therefore, to consider why they have been planned in the first place, and why they are being built now. The author of one scheme commented in a national consultation on handicapped children that he himself was opposed to it but had been ordered from higher up to produce a plan. Somewhere in the hierarchy there must be a desire for Disability Complexes, and this desire needs to be examined carefully.

Visibility: The Disability Complexes will be highly visible, both from the prestige point of view and that of demonstration. It is politically useful for the Government to be able to say to its own people: "See what a very large and impressive provision we have made for the handicapped". Like other prestige projects, they serve several purposes. They draw public attention to a facility and put it 'on the map', which is useful in the case of disabilities since the prevailing attitude is to ignore handicapped people or to put them out of sight. They boost the confidence of Government officials who are able to show foreign visitors what an impressive modern institution has been erected for the disabled. They proclaim that Pakistan is not merely a nation of peasants living in mud huts and scraping a living out of the soil. The psychological value of the prestige project should not be under-estimated; the entire development of Pakistan is crippled by lack of confidence and poor world-wide image, and prestige projects may help overcome these national handicaps. They may also give a boost to rehabilitation professionals who have for long been the cinderellas of the health, education and welfare world. Even if they are not able to secure jobs in the prestige scheme, they may feel that it indicates the dawn of official interest in their field.

So far as demonstration is concerned, if the prestige Disability Complex were in fact a 'model' to be imitated or emulated elsewhere, then the more visible the better. Compare, for example, the opposite end of the spectrum, the Community Rehabilitation scheme: however well it works in any locality, it will lack visibility and thus be more difficult to publicize and duplicate. To 'visit' a Community Rehabilitation program would mean visiting a number of homes, many of them very humble, spread out over a possibly wide area. People will not easily be impressed with it unless they already know enough about rehabilitation and development not to need to visit it. On the other hand, the prestige project may impress people, and is easy to visit. The snag, of course, is that if a project is big and expensive, it is not likely to be duplicated very widely.

Planners, and governments as a whole, like to see the results of their activity, to take pride in them, and to leave what they believe to be a worthy monument behind them. They also like to feel that they have caught hold of a problem and given it a good wallop. The grandiose building for the handicapped satisfies these inclinations. It also appears to encapsulate the problem. If one can have 100 disabled people getting treatment in one place, then why not 500 or 1,000, with all categories of handicap and every possible type of equipment, specialist, therapist, all under one roof, neatly tied together — just as they have (or are imagined to have) in America.

Models: Belief in setting up model centers has declined somewhat among Aid personnel over the past ten years or so, since it became evident that the 'model center' is almost by definition so atypical from conception through to the finished product that it can never be copied, or at any rate is very rarely copied elsewhere. However, during this period of time the term 'model center' has been much bandied about and has passed along with much other development jargon into the subconscious minds of planners in developing countries, whence it surfaces with a reflex jerk whenever something new and worthy is proposed for which scanty resources are available.

Sometimes it is confused with the phrase 'center of excellence', which is certainly a model in one sense of the word, i.e. a center which maintains very high standards to which all others may aspire; but that is scarcely a model in the other sense, i.e. a standard type which may readily be duplicated. It is not surprising that planners should fall into wishful thinking and believe that they are setting up a 'model center of excellence' which somehow, producing an abundance out of nothing, will be duplicated to produce excellence all over the place.

The realistic development model center would start with typical conditions and average staff, and aim to demonstrate that with new methods or improved techniques much better results can be obtained for the same average input. Needless to say, this rarely takes place. The temptation to load the odds in favor of success is overwhelming, even if to do so undermines the whole experiment.

The Influential: The rich and powerful in every country in whose hands (or under whose influence) are the planning and financing of projects, always have planned and presumably always will plan for the maximum benefit of the rich and powerful. It is very difficult for them to do otherwise, since the very fact of their own power and wealth limits their understanding of the world; and were they to do otherwise, they would very soon cease to be rich and powerful. However, if some benefit accrues incidentally to the masses of powerless little people, the planners are very happy. It soothes their conscience, and also serves to take the edge off the bitterness of the powerless. All across the development board, whether it is agriculture, education, health, housing or welfare, the same problem of distribution occurs. The few who have much can always arrange to be supplied with more; the many who have little tend to lose even what they have.

When it comes to rehabilitation facilities, the rich and powerful are obviously more concerned to have in their country a few prestige centers of international standard which can give first-class treatment to a small number of persons per year, than to have hundreds of modest local day-centers giving a lower standard of rehabilitation to thousands of people, or to have a home-based Community Rehabilitation scheme giving a small boost to several hundred thousand.

In the past, and still to some extent today, the wealthy have gone abroad for rehabilitative treatment for their children. However the cost of treatment in the industrialized world has become extremely high, due in part to the surge in salaries of lower grade workers in the West and the increasing differential in living standards between the 'haves' and 'have nots'. Since the salary surge has not taken place in the developing countries, it appears feasible to set up and run advanced rehabilitation facilities much more cheaply, using exploited labor in these countries. It is, therefore, no surprise to find that grandiose Disability Complexes follow hard on the heels of prestige Disease Palaces set up in major cities of Asia, despite Western advice that a more appropriate and more widely distributive scheme of health and welfare should be planned.

For Westerners to complain about this is usually hypocritical in that most Westerners would be very reluctant to accept a substantial decline in their own standard of living and enjoyment of facilities in order to share economic power with nations less well endowed. There is no more reason to expect wealthy and influential Asians to plan to give away their privileges on the national level, than to expect Westerners to do so on the international level. It is also the case that just as most Asians, so the rural handicapped and poorer urban disabled persons of Asia are invisible to the wealthier Asians. They simply do not realize that the problem is there, and in large numbers, and that the people are real flesh and blood like their own flesh and blood.

The move toward provision of residential places for the handicapped also finds some of its strongest support among the well-to-do. There would in fact be no difficulty in setting up and financing private big-city residential homes for severely handicapped persons: such homes would be over-subscribed from the first day, by families who wish to rise in career and society without the 'hindrance' of a handicapped child. Such families are not, however, good supporters of day centers. They can instead afford private tutors or nurses at home, but such measures are too slow and lack ultimate success. To them, the best solution is to pay large sums to put the child right out of their lives.

Because these families exist, are wealthy and have influence, it is practically impossible for rehabilitation to develop solely along the sort of 'appropriate' lines envisaged by western rehabilitation advisers. Even evolutionary socialist states have failed to weed out the insidious 'island of privilege' among the drab lowest-common-denominator of state services. Wealthy families will always be there offering large sums of money for specialist treatment or for residential institutions for their handicapped members. (It is a tribute to the fine character of our own Pakistani staff that several have turned down very lucrative offers of personal tutorship to the handicapped children of the rich, in order to continue working for low pay at the Mental Health Center.)

Once there are some high-level facilities in existence, any lower level of professional competence or any more demanding form of rehabilitation (like the Community Rehabilitation scheme, which throws the burden back onto the family) will be compared and contrasted and found less attractive by planners and consumers.

An incidental problem which may be foreseen in the work of the expensive, specialized rehabilitation facilities currently being planned, derives from the social class and expectations of the wealthy families who will patronize them. The sort of vocational skills and crafts acceptable by such families for their handicapped offspring are very different from those appropriate to the lifestyle of most of the population. Many mentally handicapped people, for example, can usefully and enjoyably be trained in gardening skills and other quite humble occupations. However, it is unacceptable to rich families that their child should do any such menial work, whatever its therapeutic value. Thus the wealthy families will ensure that even if some handicapped persons from poorer families manage to gain admission, the type of vocational training provided will be inappropriate.

The highly qualified: Allied with the wealthy and influential planners and Government ministers are the highly qualified medical personnel, psychiatrists and psychologists, who return to Pakistan after gaining skills and experience in the West. Whatever their motivation for returning to their country, they are often not committed agents of development, having become thoroughly westernized and determined to accept nothing below the professional and living standards to which they have become accustomed. Some are infused with an overwhelming sense of the sacrifice they are making in leaving the West, and feel that they are more than entitled to any perks they can pick up. Such people often know nothing about the living conditions of the masses in their own country. The majority of professionals who succeed in going abroad for further experience and training originate in the wealthier sections of society, which gives them the initial head start on the educational ladder in addition to the influence necessary to gain scholarships to study abroad, and the capital to set themselves up overseas. They may return with notions of doing some good to their old country, but the only thing they really know and understand is how to work the sophisticated systems of the West.

These people tend to accentuate the divorce existing between white-coated professionals and technicians in the rehabilitation world, and the lowly class of *ayas* and junior teachers who actually make physical contact with handicapped children. Nowhere is this divorce more clearly seen than in the field of physiotherapy. The art and science of massage and manipulation has a vulnerable history in the sub-continent, and is a potentially very great indigenous resource to combat physical handicap. However, the trained physiotherapists with their three-year degree of B.Sc. regard themselves as much too well-qualified to use their hands in physical contact. They are qualified to flick switches on expensive electrical machines, into which their aides and subordinates place the handicapped person. Like the bazaar psychiatrist with his electric shock machine, they are set up for life once they can acquire their own expensive gadgetry with which to carry on private practice.

Empire and ego building: As has already been implied, the personal ambitions and aspirations of planners and philanthropists play a considerable part in decisions about strategy for rehabilitation. Perhaps it is indelicate to point this out; but there is often a hint of indelicacy about the reality of rehabilitation work. Disabled people are singularly defenceless against the drives and ambitions of non-handicapped people. Both in the private and the government sectors there is a strong drive towards setting up little empires, with one supreme ego sitting in command of scurrying minions. Given a choice between enormous centralized handicap palaces, small local day-centers or home-based community rehabilitation, there is no doubt where the majority of rehabilitation professionals will cast their vote. To expect them to opt for the humble schemes which yield very low professional ego-gratification is to ignore elementary psychology.

Examples abound in Pakistan of thriving rehabilitation work being taken over by interfering busybodies, sometimes after a stiff battle, and then being maintained on paper while falling to pieces in practice. Leprosy work in the North West Frontier was taken over in this way. Work for the blind both in Karachi and Lahore has needlessly been taken over and pulled to pieces with no thought for the welfare of the handicapped persons, but purely in the enlargement of some so-called philanthropists' private empires. A school for the mentally retarded in Rawalpindi was involved in a three-year battle for control, precisely at the moment when large government grants became available. The first casualties of course, were the retarded pupils who stopped attending even as a start was made in putting up new buildings.

Even some quite well-conceived UN/Aid agency projects can be guilty of major disruption to existing rehabilitation work, by their weight and magnetism. One week before this was written, our physiotherapist was offered double his present salary to go and work with a refugee aid organization. Fortunately, the person involved was committed to his work with orthopedically impaired children and would not give it up although a higher salary was being offered. Later, we were able to negotiate for him to work in his spare time with the other agency. During the past 6 months we have had requests for our participation in various international projects, with sizeable inputs of money. The projects are good, and we need the money to maintain our own base, but we know from past experience that to go into these projects would swamp the rest of our work.

COMMUNITY REHABILITATION

It has already been pointed out that Community Rehabilitation (CR) schemes will have little appeal to the professionals. And despite some sales talk from the WHO team pushing Community Rehabilitation proposals, the scheme has no chance of success without a considerable measure of active support from rehabilitation professionals.

Nevertheless, it is quite likely that it will succeed in being launched in Pakistan in a small way, just as Primary Health Care schemes have been launched to an extremely lukewarm reception by the medical profession. Once the planners have made sure of their islands of privilege —those huge rehabilitation projects which will look after the handicapped from wealthy families—they are not against throwing a few crumbs to the rural masses in remote villages. The presentation of the WHO scheme is well adapted to reinforce this—remote village—concept, and it is being sold as a very cheap scheme, all of which appeals to planners and politicians.

The likelihood is that as long as there is foreign support coming in for the Community Rehabilitation scheme, and as long as there are free trips abroad for consultations, and a general flurry of apparent activity and money being thrown around on additional staff, planning cells, seminars, community rehabilitation officers, reports, evaluation of reports, research grants for baseline data etc., there will be vague government approval for the scheme. These initial stages can be spun out for two or three years without a single handicapped child being benefitted. However, when the initial burst of enthusiasm and foreign capital dies down, the official interest will die too. The Health and Social Welfare officials have no reason to turn down overseas assistance, as long as it lasts. The overseas agencies will try to tie up the scheme so that what they start must be carried on by the Government, but such promises are easily made, easily broken, and the break easily disguised so that overseas aid will continue to roll in for other new projects.

Instead of rushing into Community Rehabilitation, it would be better if the WHO and interested governments took a long hard look at their experience with Primary Health Care, where there is ten years worth of hard-won experience written up for the warning of future enthusiasts. The authors of the Community Rehabilitation scheme appear to have studied a certain number of PHC manuals but there is little evidence that they have also applied themselves to reading critical evaluations of PHC schemes. Yet the following problems into which PHC schemes have run in Asia will all have their equivalents in Community Rehabilitation efforts, both here and most probably in many other parts of the world.

1. Opposition from professionals in the health field, and the inertia of the status quo; in addition, there is, nowadays, an increasing strength of opposition to all schemes originating in New York, Geneva, or Stockholm.

2. Opposition from local communities, who have become suspicious of the development worker's latest ploy after two 'development decades' of bright schemes and pilot projects. Local communities are often quite well aware that if they accept a couple of PHC workers then there is no chance of getting a village hospital with doctor and nurse, whereas if they hold out for the traditional pattern they might eventually get somebody with influence to give them what they really want. (Rural folk are often in less of a hurry than Western city-based advisers.)

3. Difficulty of finding suitable front-line personnel: the ones most acceptable to the local community tend to be older, less literate, less flexible, less ready to grasp and implement the required methods, whereas the more easily trainable younger ones cut less ice in the community. The ones who do well in training and implementing the scheme naturally have career ambitions and do not expect to remain forever as voluntary or poorly paid workers at the bottom of the pyramid. In many places there are mobility restrictions on female workers, and by the same token there is no access for male workers to female clients.

4. Preventive health, hygiene and sanitation education invariably get neglected in favor of curative medicine since the latter brings quick, visible results (sometimes linked with a small financial gain from sale of drugs), whereas the former does not.

5. PHC workers need adequate supervision, back-up, encouragement, adequate referral systems, and regular refresher courses or further training, if they are to function well and retain some enthusiasm for their work. All of this requires a considerable administrative structure and competence in an area of shortage. The 'Health and Health Related Statistics' published by the Government of Pakistan for 1978 show that in rural areas 99% of the paramedical posts were filled, whereas 66% of the doctors' and 44% of the nurses' posts were lying vacant (a shortage roughly 3 times worse than that in urban areas).

In addition to problems equivalent to the above, the following difficulties are likely to be faced by CR workers:

6. There is far greater public prejudice against handicap than there is about illness. In most places there will be a tendency to conceal handicapped members of a family, partly out of shame, partly in order not to spoil the marriage chances of other members.

Thus before any rehabilitation can take place, the handicapped must be found and their families persuaded to make public their disability.

7. The PHC worker does at least treat patients directly, whereas the C.R. scheme envisages two removes: the Local Supervisor (with a few weeks training) tries to find a family Trainer (who gets a few hours orientation), while the main fount of wisdom is a manual. In most parts of the developing world there is no tradition of reading, assimilating and referring back to the printed word. Even if as many as 30% of the adult population is 'literate', less than a quarter of them are likely to have the habit of reading.

8. Families with a handicapped member come to the specialized rehabilitation facilities in the big city hoping for a cure. When we tell them that there is no cure, but that years of determined effort will very probably result in a transformation of their handicapped relative, they are often not interested. They want a cure, not hard work. If we as trained professionals fail to convince many of these families, the C.R. worker is going to be even less convincing.

9. Compared with health care, where results can show up within a few hours or days of commencing treatment, improvements are likely to be slow in C.R., and with the mentally retarded barely perceptible. Most of the retarded children we see have some degree of disturbance, and it may take 6 months or more of intensive work to overcome this. The average child takes several weeks to overcome negative behavior patterns learnt within the family. The daily escape to school provides a chance to start again at making relationships. This is of course not possible with the C.R. scheme, where it is precisely the family who do the training, though they may in fact present the greatest psychological obstacle in the initial stages.

Experience in the West of helping families to participate at home in the progress of their retarded child has shown that this is practicable only where extremely detailed child development charts are available in terms comprehensible to the parents, so that they can gain encouragement and make appropriate programs by observing the child's small forward steps. Otherwise most of their time will be wasted trying to teach the child large steps which are not possible without an understanding of the many intermediary stages. Or steps may be completely out of order, as when parents try to get their child writing the A.B.C.'s before he can discriminate between a straight line and a parabola, or manipulate a pencil. The idea that the C.R. worker should merely go on exhorting the Trainer to keep trying, for six months or more, without any visible progress before seeking the help of a specialist is naive and unrealistic. Both Trainer and C.R. worker will have become disillusioned before long, and the handicapped child will be plunged deeper into failure.

10. The lack of information and resources for rehabilitation even in Western developed countries, compared with what is available in the medical field, puts the C.R. worker at a further disadvantage. Family participation in rehabilitation on a large scale has only just begun in the West. The fact that the authors of the WHO manual seem to know so little about it is evidence of its novelty! There seems to be some danger of rushing in with the latest trend as the panacea for the rural handicapped of the developing countries.

11. Misinformation confidently given by qualified doctors, slightly garbled by the recipient and then rigidly adhered to, is also a major hazard for the C.R. worker, who will almost always have much lower status than the doctor. We have had children removed from our school because a doctor has advised parents that "nothing can be done and it is a waste of money sending the child to a special school." A deaf child came in recently whose parents had been assured by several doctors that they should not try a hearing aid until he was 12 years old. A neuro-surgeon confidently advised parents to get a baby-walker for a child who above all needed movement stimulation which the baby-walker, of course, merely hampered. The senior physician at one of the Mission Hospitals was unable to distinguish polio from cerebral palsy, and consequently, misdirected the parents. A five-minute consultation with these doctors outweighs and nullifies hours of work spread over weeks by the lowly C.R. worker.

FURTHER PSYCHO-SOCIAL FACTORS

In order to understand why the handicapped and disabled in developing countries are among the most neglected in their community and are likely to remain so for many years, it is necessary to look at the background of the whole community. The majority of handicapped persons for whom no facilities of help are available live in communities where many people have to struggle for their daily bread, or where the daily bread is fairly certain but other elements of human life with dignity are not assured. Where the majority of a community are oppressed either by physical need or fear of need, or by the grip of money-lenders, hard-faced employers and landlords, a harsh political system or by the breakdown of family systems through migration, urbanization and housing shortages, or as is commonly the case by a combination of several of these factors, there may be little or no surplus energy or compassion to spare for the weaker members of the community.

It has been discovered in may places and circumstances that until people achieve a certain freedom from want, until their more fundamental needs have been satisfied—e.g. for food and shelter, for loving care, purpose and personal recognition— and satisfied for sufficiently long that they no longer fear a rapid relapse into need, it is very difficult for them to develop altruistic feelings, to place themselves in the shoes of others, to enter into other people's suffering and make some empathetic contribution to its relief. The people who laugh when they see a cripple dragging himself/herself along, or a blind man bumping into an obstacle, are not necessarily vicious or barbaric. It is more likely that they have simply not had the opportunity to develop higher feelings, because of their own pinched circumstances.

This carries one difficult implication for the development of programs for handicapped persons in economically disadvantaged countries. Most development programs are beginning to see the need for involving village people and city slum-dwellers in planning and implementing their uplift. There is the advantage that the people work for visible benefit to themselves and their families. The whole community benefits visibly when clean water comes on tap, electricity is installed, roads are built, agricultural innovations bear fruit. In the case of the handicapped, however, there is little visible and general benefit derived from their uplift.

Average individuals with a minimal standard of living can scarcely be expected to raise much enthusiasm for participating in the program when they see no benefit for themselves and their immediate family. There will of course be some noble exceptions, those rare individuals who succeed in rising above their own personal needs and circumstances, but one cannot count on finding such people. It will be sufficient advantage if cooperation can be found even in the immediate family of the handicapped person, who at least can see some benefit and have some kinship reasons for helping to rehabilitate their disabled relative. Even this is far from automatic, especially if the disabled person is female.

For the millions of families in absolute poverty, the birth of a handicapped child (or an accident or illness resulting in a serious impairment) is a blow that puts them in a slightly worse position than their neighbors. It will probably have an adverse effect on the marriage opportunities of the rest of the family. There may be unavoidable medical expense from local quacks, in addition to the cost of travel to shrines in search of help. There is no hope that the new child might bring any upswing in the family fortunes. Therefore even the best-planned and executed rehabilitation program will have only one certain effect: the rest of the village or city slum will know for sure that this family has a handicapped member, a fact which the family may have been at pains to conceal.

Until the general level of living of the population has risen, it must be expected that the people who take any interest in the handicapped are either themselves handicapped or have attained a standard of living (both economic and emotional) sufficient for them to look around and be moved by the needs of others. This explains why at present in Pakistan, for example, most of the people actively involved in rehabilitation of the handicapped are either handicapped, or parents of handicapped children, and in both categories are quite well-to-do. The rest are mostly professionals in the health, welfare or education field who have made this their specialization for a variety of reasons. There are perhaps a few 'pure' philanthropists, and even more wealthy individuals seeking personal fulfilment and the exercise of authority in a socially praiseworthy and status-boosting occupation.

Even the above thesis is open to question, when one considers the case of the Harijans of India. Like the mentally handicapped, these casteless millions still suffer rejection and scarcely attain human status in the more backward areas, as a result of mistaken myths and religious notions. Like the mentally handicapped (who are still known in the West as 'Les Enfants du Bon Dieu') the Harijans (Children of God) are hardly accepted as children of men. This continues to be the case, though to a lesser extent than formerly, despite legislation, despite the life of Mahatma Gandhi, and the fact that at least 300 million of India's population are no longer struggling in the depths of poverty. Much of the persecution in fact comes from the wealthy and powerful landlords, and the Brahmins who though often poor are highly privileged, both groups feeling threatened from beneath by the Harijans.

Similarly, rehabilitation programs for the handicapped in very poor areas must expect to run into opposition from local people, who may feel that the 'pecking order' for outside help is being disturbed. 'The handicapped, who are little more than beggars, should come at the end of the queue for assistance.' Provision of employment skills will be resented by the able-bodied unemployed; special educational measures will be opposed by parents who cannot find a school for their normal child. Even if care of the handicapped is provided by basic health workers who also provide medical care for everyone else, it may be seen as an unwarranted intrusion into their program.

A MIDDLE WAY IN DEVELOPING REHABILITATION SERVICES

The current state of rehabilitation services throughout Asia gives little cause for satisfaction. It has been our task over the past few years to work in Peshawar running special schools and trying to understand what is happening in the rehabilitation field and how things may usefully be developed. The current appalling state of affairs serves as a spur to better planning, which must start by a clear perception of what is going on and why it is going on. There is something rather ludicrous in the fact that the government of this and other economically weak countries are planning highly specialized and professionalized, astronomically expensive big-city residential institutions, while the UN agencies with their highly paid staff are promoting cheap, rural, home-based general rehabilitation. Neither policy is likely to be used much in the next five years. The drawbacks of the government schemes are well known. The UN/WHO schemes are potentially very useful, but not until there is an adequate regional support base and sufficient surplus of professional rehabilitation skill to supervise, encourage and advise the frontline community rehabilitation workers. Without such support the Community Rehabilitation schemes will do no better than the Primary Health Care schemes in similar circumstances.

There is a middle way between the expensive institution and the home-based scheme, and it is this middle way that we are promoting in the North West Frontier Province and in some nearby parts of the Punjab. How relevant it may be to other parts of the world will depend on population distribution and the temperament of the people. It is not an ideal plan, but it has already achieved some degree of mobilization of local resources, and promises to do a good deal more.

The crucial issue is that of producing and distributing rehabilitation skills and experience from which further strategy can emerge. The grandiose government projects concentrate specialist skills in one place and on few clients. Even if they develop training courses, the training will be inappropriate for later application of skills in much reduced circumstances even supposing the practitioners are willing to go where they are needed. The Community Rehabilitation schemes attempt to disseminate a very low level of information and skills very widely, but will stumble through use of an inappropriate medium (the printed word) with inadequate reinforcement. The middle way aims at a modest but effective level of skill/experience with adequate support applied where it will have maximum usefulness. It is also open-ended both towards aiding any subsequent Community Rehabilitation scheme and towards achieveing a higher level of professional ability.

The first stage, which has already been achieved, is the strengthening of an institution to become a regional resource and training center. The Mental Health Center in Peshawar, capital of the Province, had a playground for mentally handicapped children in 1977 which was enlarged over the following three years under expatriate guidance to become a day center with 40 mentally and multiply handicapped children in attendance, a few deaf and blind pupils, a physiotherapy clinic for polio cases, and a rehabilitation and special education library. Over the past two years ten persons have received orientation courses (from 3 weeks to 4 months) with a view to setting up small schools elsewhere. The two schools have started (one in University Town, Peshawar and the other in Mardan, the second city of the Frontier). Another school is about to start, and in a fourth town plans are being made. Efforts are also being made to set up a small intermediate technology workshop to make low-cost calipers and surgical boots. There is good liaison with local government institutions for the deaf and the blind, so that their professional resources can supplement the limitations of the Mental Health Center in these handicaps.

Having established the regional base in the Provincial capital and another school in the second city, we are faced with the great mass of handicapped persons outside these cities. Certain prioritries have become apparent in our experience, guided by the general principle of doing the easy thing first. It is likely that the more visible work there is with handicapped persons, the more readily can the general public be educated and staff be trained in order to improve both quality and quantity. Doing the easy thing first maximizes the visible and successful impact of the modest initial input and gets the snowball rolling soonest. The priorities are: 1) towns before villages; 2) children before adults; 3) locally perceived needs before theoretical strategy; 4) small scale before large scale; 5) visible centers before invisible periphery; 6) well-motivated parents before indifferent families; 7) day-centers before residential work.

On this basis the easiest and most obvious thing to do is to discover well-motivated parents of handicapped children living in towns, learn from them how they perceive problems and what they would like to do about them, and steer the action towards small local day-centers. This strategy and set of priorities maximizes the likelihood of getting something viable and durable established for some handicapped children in the shortest time and at the least expense in most areas of the Frontier. If success is attained in the easiest path, more difficult ventures can then be attempted. If the easiest path proves difficult then prognosis is poor.

A project has been drawn up, with UN assistance, to fund two Rehabilitation Development Officers (RDOs) who will work full time on the mobilization of local community resources. They will start by following up families of 1,500 handicapped children already identified in a survey undertaken by degree students in 1980 in towns of 50,000 population and above in the northern half of the Frontier; a similar survey will then be conducted in the southern half of the Province. Towns of this size are spaced out across the Frontier and will eventually act as area bases for working out into surrounding rural areas (e.g. with the WHO Community Rehabilitation scheme). In a town of 50,000 there will be roughly 20,000 children aged under 16, of whom 10,000 will be boys. Experience here shows that very few girls will be brought forward regularly for rehabilitative treatment, and that only about 1% of all children are perceived as handicapped by their own community. That means about 100 boys aged under 16 in our target town. It may be possible to identify and locate half of these boys. Out of their 35 to 40 families (since some will be brothers and many cousins) it should be possible to find 3 or 4 parents who are willing to make a determined effort and contribute their own time and money jointly to provide some facilities for handicapped children. Those minimum 3 or 4 persons will be key figures with whom the RDOs will work, forming the nucleus of a Parents' Association which will register itself with the Department of Social Welfare.

What happens next will vary from place to place depending on the local flavor of the Parents' Association and their own perception and prioritization of needs. In one place they may wish to start short occupational-skill courses for older handicapped children; in another town they may decide on a morning play-ground for all handicapped children under 10. If a range of mentally retarded boys are represented, the key parents may opt for trying to start a special school for all ages of retarded children. The parents of physically disabled children might form a pressure group for an experimental integrated class at a local school for nondisabled children, and also set up an intermediate technology caliper and boot workshop. There will obviously be a good deal of conflict at this stage, as parents will inevitably be preoccupied with the needs of their own handicapped child. In some places more than one group may emerge and start separate facilities for different handicaps. It will be up to the RDOs to try to ensure that conflict is productive of action rather than anger.

Whatever the type of service decided on, the RDOs will try to steer projects toward realistic and appropriate goals relying upon local resources. Thus projects should be planned to start initially in a very modest way using someone's big room, a family's back yard, spare space in the Community Center, school rooms outside normal school hours, etc. Efforts will be made to get something going with neither the cost and delay of new buildings nor the problems of daily transport. One of the advantages of the medium-sized town is that it should be possible to find some accommodation that is adequate for a modest beginning, at little cost, and located so that a sufficient number of families will be able to bring their children by their own means of transport.

The factor which will seldom be locally available is special teaching skills. That will be suppied by the regional center giving short orientation courses (up to 3 or 4 months) to persons chosen by the Parents' Association, and possibly backing them up by the loan of an experienced teacher for a few weeks to help start things up. (This should be feasible without overburdening the regional center because developments will inevitably take place at a different rate in the 7 or 8 target towns so that the opening of day-centers will be staggered). It is anticipated that in some places parents themselves will give voluntary help; in other places there will be students fulfilling their degree requirement of practical social work, or Girls Guides, Red Crescent volunteers and so on, who will be able to assist if there is at least one person with some training who can give direction to the efforts.

The level of rehabilitation will be modest to start with, but once several small local day centers have been started it will not be difficult to arrange for the improvement of professional standards and competence. After a year or so there will be in each place perhaps half a dozen people with appreciable experience of handling handicapped children and their experience will be the base on which a tutor could build. For example, a teacher trainer could travel around, giving one day per week inservice training on a different day in each town and leaving printed material to be worked through during the following week. A summer training school could be held to consolidate this experience with a better theoretical framework. Provided that people are prepared to start small and grow at a natural pace, there should not be a great deal of difficulty getting things going, and, once started, services will not easily be stopped. Parents have greater motivation than anyone else to see something beneficial done for their handicapped child, and the greatest stamina for keeping services going.

The middle way described here is probably the easiest method of keeping the child in his normal family environment while taking some of the burden off the parents. The expensive, specialized big-city services say, 'Give us your handicapped child and we will assume the entire burden' (but they say it to extremely few); the Community Rehabilitation scheme says, 'No, he is all yours, you must keep him and help him at home.' The middle way gives the parents, especially the mothers, a break from their child and gives the child a break from his/her family, while being close enough to the home to be able to enlist family cooperation and participation. Giving the child a chance to make fresh relationships from scratch can be a very big step towards rehabilitattion. Often in addition to the initial impairment, the handicapped child suffers from intense and long-standing hang-ups within the family, due sometimes to peer-protection, under-stimulation, or other attitudes not conducive to balanced behavior. The family, too, is enabled to see the child through fresh eyes and with a new reserve of patience gathered during the spell of time that the child is out of the home.

Apart from catalysing and motivating local parents, guiding them towards realistic and appropriate goals, liaising with local health, education and welfare professionals, and coordinating the activities with the regional center, the RDOs will undertake several subsidiary projects. The need will arise for a variety of cheap, robust equipment, most of which can be made by local carpenters and metal workers if simple diagrams and measurements are provided. Written reports on progress of various aspects of their work should form the basis for a Guide and Handbook for parent groups elsewhere who wish to start their own small rehabilitation service. Training and advisory material will be produced with help from the regional center for teachers, skill instructors, parents, and local health, education and welfare professionals. Detailed child development observation and assessment charts will have to be drawn up with appropriate cultural adaptation. Simple methods must be devised and appropriate material written for training Maternal and Child Health center staff to carry out elementary hearing, sight, and mental ability testing of young children. If the RDOs have an aptitude for it they may attempt a general systems-analytical description of handicap in the towns of the North West Frontier Province, with help and guidance from the regional center, which will also provide relevant material from various parts of the world for all the above exercises.

For appropriate skills training there will need to be a study to identify common, inexpensive marketable items which require few components, simple tools and not very complicated processes, e.g. raffia fans and mats, rubber buckets and flower pots (from old tyre rubber), chicken wire, candles, twine and rope, netting, clothes pegs, gummed cardboard boxes, paper bags, various sorts of brush, simple carved toys, etc. These items should be written up from supply and cost of raw materials through the necessary tools and processes to local market outlets for the finished product. If skills centers are set up for older handicapped children they should aim within a finite time period, perhaps 6 months, to teach each child how to make at least two or three items out of a dozen or more possibilities, and then to take in a new group of handicapped children and repeat the process. This will avoid the customary decline of the vocational training center, in which the first intake of trainees stay on for many years, perhaps paying their way but preventing any turnover of trainees. Again, the level of training is not very high and the finished products may barely show a profit, but the change in social position of the young handicapped person will be considerable if he/she is able to sit at home either by himself or with other handicapped persons for company and mutual support making something of recognizable usefulness. Where it is possible for girls to get training, the elements of domestic science will probably be most appropriate, since women in the Frontier spend almost all their life at home.

The RDOs will be responsible for the introduction of creative thinking and experiments with new possibilities in vocational training. Discussion in this area so far, in Pakistan, has not got beyond the assumption that there are only two settings for economic activity by handicapped persons: either free labor market status or sheltered workshops. Publications by the International Labor Office however list more than ten times this number of types of economically useful activity which may work out in several thousand different employment situations. It will be the exacting but rewarding task of the RDOs to bring such alternatives to the attention of local Associations who are otherwise unlikely to break new ground.

Financing the above schemes from local resources should not be much of a problem. The sort of families whose attitude is to get something done for themselves rather than expecting the government to do everything for them are also the families who can find money when they want to do something. The principal running costs of the schemes envisaged will be the salary of the teacher or skill-trainer. Most of this could be met from the joint pockets of 6 or 8 average families whose handicapped children are benefitting. In fact, if certain standards are met the Education Ministry may be prepared to pay a teacher's salary, since all children have a constitutional right to education and the government is not providing appropriate schooling for the handicapped. Capital grants for equipment are not difficult to find, either from government or from larger charitable organizations—Zakat Foundation, Embassy and UN staff and so forth. Local notables and other wealthy people, banks and factories, the big pharmaceutical companies, women's organizations, and so on, will all be sources of annual donations. Services for handicapped children, once they have started and something is visibly going on, are popular objects for charitable impulses, since they have a deserving image and are non-political and non-sectarian.

UN funding for the RDOs may last two or three years, until local projects are firmly established. If government continues the project, it will at least know that it is funding a successful effort which with a modest investment pays big returns in the mobilization of local community resources. In any case, established local centers will continue with assistance from the regular Social Welfare officers posted in every town.

WHAT ABOUT THE VILLAGES?

The concern shown by some Western advisers for 'the villages of Asia' is not entirely unrealistic, though it is often romanticized and sometimes heavily colored by experience in African nations where very different social customs and systems prevail. The projects and principles described above are not done in ignorance of the fact that 80% of the population live in rural villages. Rather, they are seen as an essential preliminary step towards reaching the rural masses. On the basis of Primary Health Care experience it appears that without adequate back-up services, the Community Rehabilitation scheme envisaged by the WHO will have little success. The setting up of some rehabilitation work in the towns throughout the Frontier will provide a focus for interest and concern, and small resource bases from which Community Rehabilitation schemes could start. (The preventative and educative aspects of the WHO scheme can be going on through village development workers and health education personnel but those aspects are not strictly speaking 'rehabilitation').

Once it becomes known that something has started in the town for the handicapped, there will be families coming in from rural areas to see what is being done and to seek help for their handicapped children. In addition to on-the-spot counseling, they could be given some of the WHO material to work through, and be advised to come back after a month or so to check progress. This already happens in Peshawar, with families coming in from up to 300 miles away for advice periodically. There will be an element of self-selection in this: the families who make their way to the town will be the more highly motivated ones, who will tend also to persevere with such material and advice as they are given. When some experience has been built up in this way of parent counseling and using the WHO material, it may be possible to place the material more widely, e.g. in M.C.H. centers of surrounding rural areas, with a short orientation course for the M.C.H. center staff so that they can act as a distribution base and first point of enquiry for parents with handicapped children. Later still, on the basis of the experience gained in these ways, it may be possible to extend the service by sending out general rehabilitation aides with the WHO material (much revised and improved by this time) to contact mothers in their homes.

FUTURE STOCK NOW

The few ideas outlined above are for the most part rather obvious, and have had some success in various parts of the world at different times. However, they derive from the past and are no more than temporary expedients. Planning for the 1980s should not be confined within a framework of ideas and aspirations from the 60s and 70s. Changing social and economic conditions are rushing headlong upon the provincial towns of Asia, leaving many traditional systems high and dry, many people bewildered and fearful, many leaders on the retreat from reality, and handicapped people as usual at the end of every queue and at the bottom of every pile.

It is clear that there is insufficient political skill and will among national politicians throughout Asia to achieve the sort of redistribution and appropriate application of resources that could lead to "Primary Health Care for All by 2000 A.D.", let alone "Primary Rehabilitation for All Handicapped Persons". Just as there seems little likelihood of the wealthier nations redistributing their wealth and power in any significant degree towards the poorer nations, it is wishful thinking to imagine that the able-bodied public in Asia is going to give anything more than cosmetic aid to handicapped people. If the poorer nations and handicapped persons manage to arrive at a better position, it will be almost entirely through their own efforts.

Those of us who are concerned for the rights of handicapped persons to lead lives with some degree of human worth and dignity must consider what sort of societies are likely to exist in ten and twenty years time, and what tools or weapons we can provide to handicapped persons now to enable them to survive to battle, and to achieve worthwhile goals, in a world where less and less even of able-bodied people will obtain remunerative employment or have any real control over the circumstances of their own lives.

'Education', which used to be the panacea for a bleak future, has not been tried and found wanting, but rather has been tried and found difficult and has been substituted by 'schooling', a process of rote-learning and ideological indoctrination that is responsible for greater handicapping of the human mind and spirit than all biomedical factors and other environmental influences put together. To submit already disabled children to this stultifying practice by attempting widespread integration into the normal schooling system as it presently exists, is as little future-oriented as to add 'Molotov cocktail' to the list of common, inexpensive items which handicapped persons might be trained to make.

Welfare programs, including those for the handicapped, are certainly seen in no more favorable terms by one of the better known proponents of grass-roots development, Paulo Freire: 'They act as an anaesthetic, distracting the oppressed from the true causes of their problems. They splinter the oppressed into groups of individuals hoping to get a few more benefits for themselves' (Freire, 1972). It would be interesting to try some of Friere's adult literacy techniques for self-liberation with disabled persons. This could take place anywhere in the world, and with any of the varieties of handicap. It has been established that people learn to read very much more quickly and develop thinking and reflective capacity when the material on which they start is a matter of intense personal and political interest to them. For adult mentally retarded persons who wish to learn to read, a literacy primer should be prepared that would cover the struggles for independence of a mentally retarded person, the various trials, obstacles and psyschiatrists he or she overcomes, and the eventual triumph of independent living. Intellectually demanding equivalents are not difficult to imagine for non-literate adults with other handicaps.

Another technique which we hope to try out here in Peshawar is the use of training in thinking, decision-making, analysis and such-like mental and life skills. Since it has been established by De Bono and others that such skills can be taught, and should be taught, but are very rarely taught—certainly not in the schooling system prevailing throughout the developing world—this presents an opportunity particularly for physically disabled and blind persons (i.e. those handicapped persons who have less communication problems) to develop these skills and to use them to win a place of respect in their community. Such skills are not immediately marketable in the way that basket-weaving is, but they are rarer and more valuable and in the long run one handicapped person who has learnt, developed and begun to apply creative thinking to his own life, his family and surrounding community, should be able to outstrip any ten basket-weavers both economically and in every other sphere.

Even for the mentally retarded person it has been shown by De Bono's Cognitive Research Trust that considerable progress can be achieved and that this has a liberating effect on the person who is accustomed to failing in the usual grind of 'knowing the right answer'. When introduced to questions which have ten or more answers, the relative merits of which may be examined and kicked about, there is more opportunity for the slower thinker to gain a feeling of success and control over ideas.

Politicized literacy, access to information, creative thinking and methods of propagating ideas, all seem to have great potential for unleashing the hidden and pent-up energies of handicapped persons all over the world, and for equipping them to fight their own battles in the ever more complex muddle of clashing cultures and disintegrating social systems.

UPDATE TO DECEMBER 1984

Since 1981, when this chapter was written, there have been a number of useful developments both in Government plans and in practical achievement of the goals set out in "A Middle Way". While work has proceeded with some of the Disability Complexes, the government has also taken useful steps to strengthen existing resources of staff skills and existing non-government institutions. The Government commissioned research by the Mental Health Center into integrated education and into attitudes of the public towards disabled persons and ways to improve them. The WHO/UNICEF Community Based Rehabilitation scheme field tested in the Punjab, and the FAMH/UNICEF Community Rehabilitation Development Project in the North West Frontier, have both taken place with Government approval and interest. The work of the latter project has been consolidated and expanded during 1984 by Rehabilitation Development Officer, Mr. Sibghat-ur-Rehman. In addition to the existing centers at Peshawar and Mardan, neighborhood centers for handicapped children have opened at Mansehra, Wah Cantt., Nowshera, Mingora, Badaber, Abbottabad and Karak. Associations of parents and other interested persons have also mobilized at Dera Ismail Khan, Kohat and Charsadda, while contacts have been made for initial groundwork at Bannu, Haripur, Tank, Shabqader, and Chitral. Some of the established centers are planning to extend their services to a wider catchment area.

Project support communications activities by the Mental Health Center have produced Urdu manuals on teaching mentally handicapped pupils, elementary pediatric physiotherapy, home teaching of blind young children, vocational rehabilitation of disabled young persons, and on child development. Radio broadcasts have commenced in Puhsto aimed at basic rural rehabilitation at the village level.

The Coordinator of the WHO/CBR field testing in the Punjab, Mr. Rafiq Jaffer, visited the FAMH/UNICEF project and wrote subsequently:

> *I can say with sincerity that it was a learning experience for all of us, one which will have its impact on the development of rehabilitation programs for disabled people in the Punjab. You and your colleagues are not only doing pioneering work in the rehabilitation field, but you have set up a model for community rehabilitation which works in Pakistan. And there are not*

many success stories in community work in this country. If I try to analyze why your scheme worked where others have failed, I see it as a result of a combination of factors: 1) a thorough understanding of the culture, social system and administrative set-up of the North West Frontier Province; 2) a proper analysis of the causes of failure of similar schemes in Pakistan and other underdeveloped countries; 3) the setting up of an intelligent and pragmatic strategy on the basis of points 1 and 2 above; 4) a strong faith in the ability of people to solve their own problems, given the right opportunity; 5) availability to the people of an inspiring model epitomizing the "give away to the people" attitude; 6) sheer hard work; 7) no vested interest. Obviously, the combination is rare, hence the low rate of success stories. If a similar program is to succeed in other areas, it will require most of these elements, though it will have the advantage of an available and tested strategy.

CONCLUSION

Over a period of 6 years, mobilization of local community resources for rehabilitation has taken place effectively in 12 major towns of the North West Frontier which are the foci for a settled population of about 10 million people in an area of 60,000 sq. km. This mobilization resulted from re-orienting an institution as an outgoing resource base, and then contacting and activating an already self-motivated group, i.e. close relatives of disabled children in towns. The strategy has been to "do the easy thing first" and to do it with little expense. The positive results of this low-cost exercise taking place in a difficult and less developed region suggests that similar strategies could successfully be attempted on a much wider scale in parts of Asia and Africa having comparable social and population structures.

References

Dixon, J. (1981). The welfare of the handicapped in the Peoples' Republic of China. *Journal of Rehabilitation in Asia, October.*

Freire, P. (1972). *Pedagogy of the oppressed.* New York: Herder and Herder.

8

COMMUNITY-ORIENTED PHYSIOTHERAPY FOR POLIO AFFECTED CHILDREN: A BRIEF REPORT FROM PAKISTAN

Farhat Rashid[1]

STRATEGY

A physiotherapy clinic was started in 1981 at the Mental Health Center, Peshawar, as an extension of existing special education and counseling facilities, with orientation toward mobilizing community resources for rehabilitation. The clinic was developed using simple, low-cost methods of treatment in which parents or other family members of the disabled child participated. Next, several outstations were established, employing physiotherapy assistants trained at the base clinic. A low-cost caliper workshop was added in 1982 after two of the physiotherapy assistants took a six-week course at the I.C.R.C. Paraplegic Centre. They now fabricate simple calipers, crutches and walkers, and make shoe raisings to compensate leg shortening.

Nearly 90% of the children examined have post polio paralysis. The remaining 10% have cerebral palsy, club foot, flat foot, post plaster stiffness of joints, etc. In practice, a physiotherapy assistant with 4 months intensive training can handle 80% of the cases encountered at outstations. Where there are complications or problems of assessment, the child is referred to Peshawar or is seen by the physiotherapist on her next visit.

In the past three years assessment tours have been made to 10 towns of the North West Frontier Province, examining 840 polio affected children. Physiotherapy assistants have been trained and outstation clinics have started under local committee supervision in 5

[1]This report was written in October, 1984.

towns: Abbotabad, Mingora, Mardan, Nowshera, and Badaber. Trainees from Karak are now undergoing training and there are plans to open centers in other towns. The local committees mostly consist of parents who are strongly motivated. Those parents whose children have been treated successfully are able to motivate families whose children are beginning treatment.

TREATMENT METHODS

Methods consisting of wax application, massage, and directed exercises are taught to the physiotherapy assistants and to family members. Wax is melted and allowed to cool to about 44°C. It is poured into a piece of polythene sheet (plastic) spread on a rectangular frame. The sheet with wax is then wrapped around the affected part of the body and enclosed in blanket or towel for about 10 to 20 minutes. After removal, massage and exercises are given over a period of one hour, including use of locally made apparatus such as parallel bars and moving weights. Walking supports such as plaster splints, wrist splints, and occasionally plasters for minor contractures are made. Patients needing surgical treatment are referred to the big hospitals. In such cases, pre- and post-surgical physiotherapy treatment is also given.

OBSERVATIONS AND RESULTS

These results were recorded at our Peshawar base clinic. Results at the outstations have been similar; the majority of polio cases occurred within the first two years of life. No case with a history of occurrence of polio later than 5 years of age was seen. Males predominated, representing 65% of cases. Lower limbs were affected more than upper limbs, and the extensor group of muscles were more involved than the flexor group.

Patient data

The number of registered polio patients stands at 340 (224 males and 116 females). There are 55 patients under treatment at the Peshawar clinic; 20 of these visit the clinic weekly and another 20 visit fortnightly, while the remaining 15 visit monthly. So far 30 polio patients have been referred for operation. Table 1 presents an age distribution of the 340 registered polio cases.

Table 1. Distribution by Age at Which Polio Occurred

Years	0 - 1	1 - 2	2 - 3	3 - 4	4 - 5	Over 5
Cases	130	172	25	7	6	Nil

Table 2. Categories of Limb Involvement

Limb Affected	Patients	%
Lower limbs: Right leg	99	29.1
Lower limbs: Left leg	93	27.3
Both legs	120	35.3
Upper limbs: right arm	1	0.3
Upper limbs: Left arm	2	0.6
Both arms	2	0.3
Right arm and left leg	2	0.6
Left arm and right leg	1	0.3
Both legs and right arm	3	0.9
Both legs and left arm	5	1.5
Right leg and right arm	6	1.8
Left leg and left arm	6	1.8

Table 3. Results and Criteria of Recovery

Group	Criteria	Patients	%
Good	Patient can walk without caliper, slight muscle weakness, +normal gait.	102	35.5
Fair	Patient can walk without caliper. Moderate muscle wasting, +abnormal gait	60	20.9
Poor	Patient can walk only with caliper. Marked muscle wasting, +abnormal gait	113	39.4
Nil	Patient can't walk even with caliper. Marked wasting. Unable to do simple work with hands	12	4.2

Limbs and muscles involved

Among the 340 polio patients, 312 (91.7%) had involvement of lower limbs only; 23 (6.7%) had involvement of both upper and lower limbs; 5 (1.5%) had only upper limbs involved. These are further categorized in Table 2. In the lower limbs, extensor of hip, knee, and dorsi-flexors of ankle were involved most. In the upper limbs, muscles around the shoulder were involved most, and muscles acting on wrist were least involved.

Duration and success of treatment

Most of the cases showed progress, i.e. return of power and restoration of function in partially affected muscle, following two to six months of simple treatment. This duration is similar to the period usually required with sophisticated methods of hospital treatment. The durations of treatment for 287 patients were as follows: 1 month—17 patients; 2 to 4 months—174 patients; 4 to 6 months—74 patients; 6 to 8 months—22 patients. The recovery results and the criteria for determining recovery are summarized in Table 3.

SUMMARY AND CONCLUSION

In polio cases in the convalescent stage, immediately after the spasm is over, active treatment with simple low-cost methods can give satisfactory results. The extension of these methods, through physiotherapy assistants working at outstations and involving family members in the treatment, can greatly increase the availability of treatment to those for whom it would otherwise be geographically and financially impossible.

PART TWO: EDUCATION—CURRICULUM DESIGN, ASSESSMENT, AND STATUS OF SPECIAL EDUCATION

9

EARLY EDUCATION CURRICULUM DESIGN FOR HANDICAPPED CHILDREN IN DEVELOPING COUNTRIES

David Baine

In the absence of sufficient numbers of specialized personnel, and adequate funds to finance costly research and development projects, there has been a tendency among developing nations to adopt curricular, instructional, and assessment procedures and material developed in western countries. Given these constraints, the approach has been economically sound. However, there are some serious educational disadvantages. The following discussion reviews some of these disadvantages, suggests ideal methods of developing ecologically valid curricula for handicapped children in developing countries, and suggests means of implementing these methods.

PROBLEMS

A number of problems are associated with the adoption by developing countries of assessment and curriculum materials based on western schedules of child development. These schedules describe the average rate, sequence, and type of development of average western children raised in average western environments. Do these schedules represent a suitable standard for judging the development of normal functioning among children in developing countries? Perhaps because of the unique nature of some of these developing environments, and the influence of experience on child development, children in these environments may develop some skills not required in western countries, and fail to develop other skills that are common to the western environment, but not required in the developing environment. An instructional program based on the developmental sequence of one geographic, cultural environment may teach skills that are of little or no functional value in another environment, while failing to to teach skills that are essential to that environment. Thus, *normal* functioning children compared to the developmental standards established for another culture may be judged at a disadvantage. Consequently, it is important that both tests and curricula be ecologically and functionally valid in the environment in which they are to be used.

For *handicapped* children in developing countries curricula based on Western schedules of child development may be even less suitable than they are for normal functioning children. Handicapped individuals, in Western countries frequently deviate quite significantly from normal developmental sequences (White & Haring, 1978; White 1980a,b). Variations may occur in terms of the number, nature, sequence, and duration of each developmental stage. For example, Adelson and Fraiberg (1974) observed that children blind from birth, when compared to normal functioning children, exhibited a delay in the acquisition of some behaviors, failed to acquire others, resequenced the order in which some skills were learned, and acquired some unique compensatory behaviors. Similarly, Guess, Sailor, and Baer (1976) noted that severely handicapped individuals radically departed from the normal pattern of development in their acquisition of speech and language skills.

If instructional sequences strictly conform to the normal sequence of development, several difficulties may arise. For instance, when a mentally retarded individual is taught skills that relate to his/her mental rather than chronological age, such skills are not functionally related to his/her current environmental demands. Children may become quite proficient with pegboards, and puzzles, and may not exhibit any improvement in their performance of functional skills.

When remediation focuses on a child's mental age level, the child will not only remain behind the development of his/her chronological age peers, but his/her development will fall even further behind. Alternatively, it is possible to develop curricula that teach chronological, age-appropriate, and functional behaviors. For example, rather than provide severely retarded adolescents and young adults with tasks appropriate to their mental age level, Brown, Branston, Hamre-Nietupski, Pumpian, Certo and Gruenwald, (1979) successfully taught functional skills like food preparation, telephone use, shopping, bus riding, and vocational skills (Snell, 1983).

Developmental approaches to instruction frequently lead to the teaching of isolated skills like *grasping* taken from the motor domain of development (Snell,1983). The skill of grasping is often not taught as an integral part of the functional task existing in the individual's current or future environment. As a result, although the student may learn to grasp in the desired manner under artificial instructional conditions, the skill may not transfer to the general environments where different conditions may exist, and where slight modifications in the behavior may be required. Thus, because of the subsequent disuse of the grasping response, it may not be retained in the student's repertoire. Failure to maintain the skill may lead some practitioners to the conclusion that it is not worth the time, effort and cost of teaching handicapped children. This conclusion would be tragic in an economically deprived environment where effective habilitation of handicapped individuals, although relatively expensive, may be of considerable economic, social and personal advantage. In fact, had the grasping response been integrated into one or more functional skills that the student could frequently perform in a rewarding manner in his/her daily life, the probability of retaining the skill would be significantly increased. Brown et al. (1979) have suggested that rather than develop curricula on the basis of performance domains such as sensory, motor, communication, and cognition, leading to the teaching of generic, isolated skills, one should define curriculum domains in terms of the demands of current and future family, community, recreational, school, vocational, and occupational environments. This procedure would ensure that curricula were comprised of functional skills.

Normative developmental schedules, tests, and curricula are derived on the basis of a cross-sectional analyses of what normal children, under the usual range of conditions, are typically capable of performing at various age levels. Developmental schedules are not derived in a top-down, task analytic approach where one identifies the essential knowledge and skills required of children at various age levels; neither are these skills task-analyzed to determine the minimum prerequisite subskills, or ordered according to their sequence of development.

As a result of this cross-sectional approach in which normative developmental schedules are developed, they may not list all of the skills prerequisite to normal development. In addition, the schedules may list a number of nonessential, but commonly found skills such as bead stringing, and block design. Activities of this nature may teach generic skills like pincer grasp, eye-hand coordination, color and shape discrimination; however, acquisition of these skills frequently does not result in an improvement of more essential functional skills of which the generic skills are a part. The research is replete with examples demonstrating that improvement in generic skills does not transfer automatically to an improvement in related functional skills (see Stokes and Baer, 1977 for a review of the literature on generalization).

When teaching handicapped children, teachers must insure that the instructional sequence contains all and only the skills necessary for development. As Becker, Engelmann and Carnine (Carnine, 1979) have demonstrated with the DISTAR reading, language and arithmetic programs, when instruction is based on task analyzed sequences and direct instructional procedures, it is possible for mentally retarded students to learn more than one year of academic growth during one year of instruction. When instruction does not teach one skill (**A**) prerequisite to acquisition of a number of other skills (**B**) within a particular area of performance, a child not only fails to learn the set of **B** skills, but also fails to learn the larger set of skills (**C**) for which the set of **B** skills were prerequisite. Children who fall farther and farther behind in a specific area of learning are often referred to as having a specific learning disability. In fact, the problem may actually exist not in the child, but in an inadequate curriculum or in inadequate instructional procedures that have failed to teach the child one essential skill.

The relative consistency of the age and sequence at which normal functioning children achieve the developmental milestones is sometimes interpreted as evidence of the basic constitutional nature and unalterable sequence of development. However, if the model of normal development is based upon the observation of normal children living within the average range of conditions, the observed developmental consistency may, to a large extent, be a function of the similarity of the nature of the experiences these children have received.

To believe that the consistency arises primarily from the basic constitutional nature of children helps to insure that retarded children remain retarded. For example, the constitutional approach is frequently associated with the concept of readiness that dictates that a child must be of mental age six before he/she is ready to learn to read. Thus, a child of IQ 50 would have to wait until chronological age 12 before the commencement of reading instruction. During the period of waiting, valuable instructional time may be lost, and at age 12, there may be other instructional priorities with little time left for reading instruction.

On the other hand, if one believes that the nature of a child's experience greatly influences the rate, type and sequence of his/her development, then rather than wait for maturational readiness, one may intervene to teach the child any skills for which the prerequisite skills exist. For example, Hayden and Dmitriev (1975), Hayden and Haring (1977), and Clunies-Ross (1979) adopted this approach when they taught Down's syndrome children to read before age six.

GOALS FOR CURRICULUM DESIGN

The general goal of curriculum design is to develop an ecologically valid curriculum that lists, in order of prerequisites first, all of the essential functional skills that will permit each handicapped student to fulfill as much and as well as possible, the common daily demands of the various environments within which he/she participates now and in the future. Because of the heterogeneity of subcultures within many developing nations, to establish ecological validity, curricula must be developed to accommodate urban, rural, and regional differences within each country. A number of guidelines are listed below that will help to achieve the general goal.

a) A curriculum must prepare students for both current and future environments in which they do or will participate. Curriculum designers must anticipate increasing demands that will be placed on individuals as a result of increases in the number of environments in which they will be involved, changes in the nature of their involvement, as well as changes within each developing environment. The curriculum designer must also identify the skills prerequisite to fulfilling the changing demands placed upon the individual. These considerations are particularly important in developing countries where current or future technological, economic and social changes may result in significant environmental modification. Also, in some developing countries where migration from rural to urban environments occurs, radical changes in demands may be made upon the individual.

b) A curriculum must include skills that will permit each learner to function optimally in family and domestic, community, recreational, school, and vocational/occupational environments.

c) A comprehensive curriculum should incorporate the instruction of motor, sensory, communication, social-personal, and self-help skills into activities that are functional in a learner's natural environments.

d) A curriculum should be designed to teach each learner skills that will permit, as much as possible, age-appropriate normative, independent functioning in the least restrictive manner in each of the environments described above.

e)The curriculum should be as economic and efficient as possible including the minimum essential skills organized so that all prerequisite skills are taught first, and excluding all nonessential skills.

f)Related to efficiency, each curriculum should adopt a direct instructional approach in which each skill is taught directly in the form and under the conditions in which it is eventually expected to be performed. This approach avoids the difficulties commonly associated with the failure of generic cognitive, perceptual, and sensory skills to transfer to specific functional skills.

g) Well designed curricula should also incorporate provisions for systematically distributing practice of acquired skills to insure maintenance of learning. Maintenance of learning refers to the ability of a learner to continue to perform a skill, as and when required, for extended periods of time, after the skill was initially learned. Like generalization, maintenance of a learned skill is frequently not automatic. To enhance maintenance of learning, curricula should provide for systematically distributed practice of newly acquired skills after successively longer periods of time. This procedure progressively lengthens the interval following which the individual must recall the skill. The interval between successive practice sessions should be as short as necessary to insure adequate recall of the skill, but as long as possible to insure retention over the longest period possible. How long any interval should be, and how rapidly intervals may be lengthened, can only be determined in terms of a particular individual and task. In successive practice sessions, the skill may also be integrated with other skills, or be performed under various conditions to promote generalization.

h) A curriculum should incorporate a criterion referenced approach in which testing is an integral part of teaching. When testing is integrated into the ongoing process of teaching, students who experience difficulty may be identified as soon as an error occurs, and appropriate correction procedure may be immediately implemented. When testing and teaching are separate activities, errors may go unnoticed for a long period of time. Unfortunately, when testing and teaching are separated, and response errors are not readily observed, children who experience difficulty with the curriculum, often receive more practice performing the wrong responses than they do performing correct responses. Short-term clinical testing outside of an instructional environment also has its problems. The shortness of the test, the atypical nature of the testing environment, and the variability of performance of many handicapped learners decrease the validity and reliability of clinical testing. On the other hand repeated observations of the usual variations in a student's performance under typical variations in instructional conditions increases the reliability and validity of the assessment.

These guidelines describe steps leading towards the development of an ideal curriculum, one that in its entirety is not often found even in western countries. Because of financial constraints, and lack of sufficient numbers of suitably trained personnel, it may be difficult to develop curricula of this nature in most developing countries. Some characteristics of the ideal may be readily achieved in some circumstances, others may be approximated to various degrees, while still others may become long-term goals. Since all curricula should be involved in a continuous process of evaluation and improvement, it is important to define the ideal toward which the curricula may evolve. The following paragraphs describe a number of procedures that assist the development of many of the ideal curriculum characteristics. Because of the limitations of the present context, and the complexity of these procedures, the discussion must of necessity be introductory. Additional sources of information are indicated.

ECOLOGICAL INVENTORY

Brown et al. (1979) have described a method of curriculum development called the ecological inventory. The purpose of this approach is to develop a curriculum comprised of functional skills that are required in a student's contemporary and/or future life spaces and that permit the individual to function as normatively, age-appropriately, and independently as possible in the least restrictive environment. The steps involved in an ecological inventory are as follows:

- A survey is conducted to identify the current and future least restrictive environments in which a handicapped individual is or can function. A study is made of the following environments: a) family and domestic, b) community, c) recreation, d) school, and e) vocational/occupational.
- Sub-environments within each area are identified. For example,

community sub-environments may include the village well, the market...

- Then the tasks within each sub-area are listed; for example, one of the tasks related to the market may include, selection of the correct type, quality and quantity of food.
- In the final stage, the skills required to perform each of the tasks are identified through the process of task analysis. These skills are then organized into instructional sequences or curricula. This process insures that all the skills necessary for functioning are included in the instructional program.

TASK ANALYSIS

A task analysis involves three concurrent activities. A particular task identified in the ecological inventory is subjected to (a) performance, (b) conditions, and (c) standards analyzed to identify the minimum essential skills prerequisite to performing the task in a satisfactory manner.

In a performance analysis, a number of novice and accomplished performers are observed performing the task under a variety of naturally occurring conditions. This analysis helps to (a) identify various methods by which accomplished performers complete the task, (b) select the simplest method of performing the task, and (c) identify common errors made by novice performers. Thus, instruction may be designed to teach the simplest method of performing while avoiding commonly occurring errors of performance.

The analysis of conditions is designed to indicate the most commonly encountered difficult conditions and the usual range of influential conditions for the purpose of teaching the learner to respond appropriately to the conditions that he/she will most likely encounter in current and future environments. The purpose of the standards analysis is to identify the minimum essential standards of performance required to perform in a normative manner in the least restrictive environment. It is especially important with handicapped learners to establish the minimum essential standards of performance so as to determine when to advance to the next level of instruction. The goal with slow learners is to advance instruction as soon as skills prerequisite to the next level of instruction have been mastered, and neither to advance instruction prematurely to failure at the next level, nor to retard development unnecessarily.

For each skill identified in the task analysis, an instructional objective is written to describe an observable, measurable behavior that a learner will perform, under the range of commonly found conditions, to the minimum essential standards to indicate mastery of the skill. These instructional objectives are then organized into instructional sequences in a curriculum. A brief instructional objective follows. Objectives of this nature serve as both the end toward which instruction is directed, and as an objective test of the success of the instruction. Thus, teaching and testing are incorporated into an ongoing process in the classroom.

> CONDITIONS: Given thirty addition problems, randomly mixed with an equal number of substraction problems, where each addition problem has two single digit addends in a vertical format, and the sum is less than or equal to eighteen.
>
> PERFORMANCE: the learner will write the correct sum,
>
> STANDARDS: of at least twenty-six of the problems in an eight minute interval on five trials randomly distributed over one month following instruction of this type of addition problem. No subtraction problems should be added. No systematic error should be made in the addition problem.

There is research evidence to indicate that when effective instructional techniques are employed to teach a curriculum that includes all of the essential skills, mentally retarded children can acquire more academic skills in one year of instruction than the average child taught with traditional methods acquires in the same period of time (Carnine, 1979).

STEPS TO APPROXIMATING THE IDEAL CURRICULUM

Where initially necessary because of limitations in funding and personnel, normative developmental sequences derived from an analysis of normal functioning western children may be adopted on an interim basis. In doing so, one should be fully aware of the potential inappropriateness of the schedule to both normal functioning and handicapped persons due to the failure to establish ecological validity, and to inadequate methods of skill sampling. Over time, all or parts of the sequence may be made more ecologically valid following the completion of ecological inventories. In later stages of development, progressively more sections of the schedule may be replaced with skill sequences derived from the task analysis of skills identified in the ecological inventory.

The *Reading Mastery* program developed by Engelmann and Bruner (1983) is based on task analysis, and has been experimentally validated on a number of different populations of learners. Although the program is ecologically invalid for use in developing countries, because of its carefully designed structure, instructional material, and empirically derived instructional techniques, the program would serve as an excellent example for the development of curricula in developing countries where there may be few highly trained teachers.

The following questions should be asked of any curriculum whether adopted from another culture, or specially designed for a particular population of learners in a particular culture.

- Are all the skills included in the curriculum essential?
- Will each of the skills, in the form in which they are taught, permit the learner to fulfill directly one or more of the common functional demands of the natural environment?
- If for particular skills, the answer to the previous question is "No", are the particular skills components of, or developmental prerequisites to, other functional skills?
- Does the curriculum contain all of the necessary and sufficient prerequisite skills to prepare the student to meet the common functional demands of the current or future environments he/she may encounter?
- Does the curriculum include the teaching of compensatory skills that may be required by handicapped individuals incapable of performing some tasks in the usual manner?
- Has the validity of the curriculum been established for the paricular type of students for which it is intended to be used?

References

Adelson, E. & Fraiberg, S. (1974). Gross motor development in infants blind from birth. *Child Development, 6*, 114-245.

Brown, L., Branston, M., Hamre-Nietupski, S., Pumpian, I., Certo, N., & Gruenwald, L. (1979). Strategy for developing chronological age-appropriate and functional curricular content for severely handicapped adolescents and yound adults. *Journal of Special Education, 13*, 81-90.

Carnine, D. (1979). Direct instruction: A successful system for educationally high-risk children. *Journal of Studies and Curriculum, 11*, 29-45.

Clunies-Ross, G. (1979). Acceleration of the development of Down's Syndrome infants and young children. *Journal of Special Education, 13* 169-177.

Engelmann, S. & Bruner, E. (1983). *Reading mastery.* Chicago: Science Research Associates.

Guess, D., Sailor, W., & Baer, D. M. (1976). *Functional speech and language training for the severely handicapped, Part I and II.* Lawrence, Kansas: H and H Enterprises.

Hayden, A. H., & Dmitriev, V. (1975). The multidisciplinary preschool program for Down's syndrome children at the University of Washington Model Preschool Center. In B.Z. Friedlander, G. M. Sterritt, & G. E. Kirk (Eds.), *Exceptional Infant, Vol. 3: Assessment and intervention.* Baltimore: University Park Press.

Hayden, A. H. & Haring, N. G. (1977). The acceleration and maintenance of developmental gains in Down's syndrome school-age children. In P. Mittler (Ed.), *Research to practice in mental retardation, Vol. 1: Care and intervention.* Baltimore: University Park Press.

Snell, M. (Ed.), (1983). *Systematic instruction of the moderately and severely handicapped (2nd Ed.).* Columbus, OH: Charles E. Merrill.

Stokes, T. F., & Baer, D. M. (1977). An implicit technology of generalization. *Journal of Applied Behavior Analysis, 10*, 349-367.

White, O. R. (1980a). Adaptive performance objectives: Form versus function. In W. Sailor, B. Wilcox, & L. Brown (Eds.), *Methods of instruction with severely handicapped students.* Baltimore: Paul H. Brookes.

White, O.R. (1980b). Child assessment. In B. Wilcox & R. York (Eds.), *Quality educational services for the severely handicapped: The federal investment.* Washington, D.C.: Bureau of Education for the Handicapped.

White, O. R. & Haring, N. G. (1978). Evaluating educational programs serving the severely and profoundly handicapped. In N. G. Haring, & D. D. Bricker (Eds.), *Teaching the severely handicapped (Vol. 3).* Seattle, WA: American Association for the Education of the Severely and Profoundly Handicapped.

10

THE DESIGN OF A BASIC ASSESSMENT CHART FOR USE WITH THE MENTALLY RETARDED IN SRI LANKA

John M. Hughes

INTRODUCTION

It is becoming apparent that even though considerable use is made of sophisticated psychometric instruments, there is considerable unease and a turning away from the traditional psychometric approach to different methods of assessing mentally retarded and other handicapped children. The ability to use informal criterion-referenced devices to measure skills is a competency expected of any good teacher (Carr, 1981; Gardner, Murphy, & Crawford, 1983; Jeffree & Cheseldine, 1983; Jeffree & McConkey, 1976; Kiernan & Jones, 1977; Simon, 1981; Whelan & Speake, 1979). Furthermore, many standardized tests are being misused in the educational assessment of non-achieving children. Few would deny their value when they are used to gather descriptive information about the general learning characteristics of groups of children, since that information serves to increase understanding of the complex phenomena related to learning. However, these tests have been criticized because they compare the mentally retarded person with an inappropriate peer group. Furthermore, the results may not lead to a teaching program, and they may not be understood because of limited and outdated concepts of intelligence.

The main reason why the findings of these tests cannot be related to a teaching program is because the test items are not, generally, selected because of their practical value in developing a person's current practical skills. What can developing countries learn from a change of approach to assessment—countries that have not fully developed their own psychometric instruments based on their own cultures, but are experimenting with such instruments in assessment of handicapped children?

One conclusion is the importance attached to the contribution that teachers can make to the comprehensive assessment of children. A profile of a child's skills and disabilities cannot easily be drawn without the observations of teachers; their systematic observations of the behavior of a child in a special group, and of the child's response to learning situations, are critical to any decision on present educational needs and the treatment required. Mittler (1979a) places particular stress on this point when he suggests that teachers should not think of assessment as a 'highly specialized set of rituals' which can only be performed by psychologists; on the contrary, assessment is essentially a task for those who are going to teach the child, whether they are teachers or parents. Therefore, assessment is not just a matter of using certain intelligence tests, but involves an attempt to establish what the child can and cannot do, with the aim of setting a teaching goal that is related to his/her immediate needs. This means that assessment defines the entry point to the curriculum. The teacher can make use of checklists that can help to pinpoint the stage that a child has reached in critical areas of development—for example, in physical development, self-help skills, play, social maturity, language and communication abilities, and so on.

However, charts and assessment scales are obviously not enough and they should be supplemented by careful and detailed observation of the child's behavior in a variety of structured and unstructured situations. Therefore, it becomes apparent that teachers in the developing countries require advice on the need to devise a simple system of recording which can be used to plan their teaching and as a means of evaluating progress. In this respect, the model provided by Gardner et. al. (1983) is extremely useful.

RATIONALE BEHIND THE DESIGN OF A BASIC ASSESSMENT CHART

Assessment should be regarded as the basis of any educational program for the mentally retarded. If we are to make a correct estimate of the individual's needs, we must know his strengths and weaknesses. Moreover, we should regard assessment as an integral part of the education of the retarded individual rather than regard assessment for assessment's sake. In other words, assessment should always be linked to a program which is designed to help the individual make some progress, however small this progress may be.

The initial assessment of a mentally retarded individual should be supported by systematic observations which are regularly recorded. It is because the mentally retarded do not always perform consistently that continuous assessment is required.

Initial assessment should highlight an individual's strengths and weaknesses over as many aspects of development as possible. More detailed information on the precise nature of an individual's difficulties can be obtained by using a more detailed assessment by means of task analytic procedures. This should arise through the actual teaching of the person because assessment and teaching are so closely related.

If one is able to break down a target skill into its constituent sequential sub-skills, then this provides the teacher with the possibility of a more detailed analysis of what the person can or cannot do. This is when the teacher will consider how he/she can plan a program which will assist the person in mastering the next sub-skill required in the series which will, it is hoped, eventually culminate in the acquisition of the target skill. It was stressed, however, that it is important to remember that an essential factor in assessing a person's level of skills is the degree of prompting required. For example, it is likely that a mentally retarded person can drink from a container if he/she is assisted with a physical prompt. Therefore, instead of saying 'No, the person cannot drink from a container', we should say 'Yes, the person can drink from a container, if a physical prompt is given'.

There was a dearth of psychometric instruments and developmental scales in Sri Lanka. However, the author hoped to make some contribution, however small, to the assessment of the mentally retarded in this country (Hughes, 1977; 1981). He was extremely fortunate to have the assistance of 15 mature postgraduate students who were members of the course which he had designed and established at the University of Colombo. The construction of the Basic Assessment Chart was an integral part of the course and arose quite naturally from the author's lectures on child development and its deviations. During the course, there was much discussion of the following assessment procedures:

- The Progress Assessment Chart (Gunzburg, 1974).
- The Portage Guide to Early Education—Checklist (CESA 12, 1975).
- PIP Developmental Charts (Jeffree & McConkey, 1976).
- The Behavior Assessment Battery (Kiernan & Jones 1977).

One aspect of the course was the completion of a child study. This work was carried out during weekly visits to a home/school where the student would be placed for 7 weeks of teaching practice. Therefore, the development of the Basic Assessment Chart was just one aspect of the preparation of materials for the child study.

A perusal and discussion of the four assessment procedures and the rationale behind the designs resulted in the obvious comment that there were many items contained in the scales that were not applicable to the vast majority of individuals in Sri Lanka. The following items are rather obvious examples of this observation, but they do reflect the difficulty of the task confronting the student:

Ties shoelaces
Cleans shoes adequately when told to do so
Stabs food with fork and brings to mouth
Puts on socks
Puts on shoes
Climbs on lavatory seat
Uses grill on cooker
Uses a vacuum cleaner
Uses washing machine
Runs bath water in preparation for a bath

The students decided to use Gunzburg's four main headings: Self-help, Communication, Socialization, and Occupation, and it was further agreed that the skills which the students were to assess were those skills regarded as essential if the mentally retarded child were to become as socially competent as possible. Furthermore, the skills should be regarded as essential 'life skills' necessary for the child to live independently within the community. This was based on the premise that all teaching should prepare the mentally retarded child to be an efficient human being (as far as this is possible) when he/she becomes an adult. Furthermore, it was agreed that academic skills (reading, writing and number) should be taught only to the extent necessary to serve the aims of social competence. Since the students were beginning to appreciate that most of the academic education is beyond the grasp of the mentally retarded, emphasis was put on a functional educational program which would help them directly to live and work in the community.

It was accepted that even though the skills contained in the Basic Assessment Chart would appear limited and deal only with the essentials, it was not being suggested that all mentally retarded children can and must achieve success in all areas and at all levels. Furthermore, it was also accepted that certain mentally retarded individuals would be able to achieve a higher level in certain academic skills but that in an educational program, basic skills would be taught first and other academic skills would be added only after these basic skills had been adequately mastered. As a result of this general discussion, one was able to move on to a discussion of the rationale behind the four areas of social growth which were to be used in the design of the Basic Assessment Chart.

THE CONTENT OF THE BASIC ASSESSMENT CHART

The 15 students were divided into four groups (3 groups of 4 and one group of 3). Each group was given the responsibility of devising skills for one of the four areas:

Group A - Self-help skills
Group B - Communication skills
Group C - Socialization skills
Group D - Occupational skills

It was agreed that the Basic Assessment Chart should be designed for use with children who were mentally retarded according to the four classifications, i.e. mildly, moderately, severely and profoundly. The completed chart would reflect an enormous range of ability in social growth. Furthermore, because the majority of mentally retarded children would not be identified or assessed until they started school at age 6, it was decided that the prime purpose of the chart would be to assess mentally retarded children between the chronological ages of 6 and 16 years.

The four groups were required to study the skills used in the four assessment procedures and select those that were applicable to their own area of study. Furthermore, the validity of their selections would be tested during their early visits to homes/schools for the purpose of preparing a child study. The class teachers were asked to participate and all the students reported that this was of inestimable value. This meant that after eight visits, or eight weeks, the four groups were ready to meet together to discuss the Basic Assessment Chart as an entity. The author served as an adviser to the four groups and acted as an arbitrator on occasions when members of the group could not agree on the selection of certain skills.

It was regarded as essential that, as far as possible, the skills should be placed in order of maturational development. In this respect, the students were encouraged to study the four assessment procedures which indicate the maturational order of the skills. Furthermore, it was emphasized that the results of the Basic Assessment Chart would be used to devise individual educational programs based on the diagnosis of specific weaknesses and the use of task analysis.

It has already been stated that some skills contained in the four assessment procedures were not applicable to children (and adults) living in Sri Lanka. However, most of the skills were applicable and relevant. Minor modifications were made in many cases. For example:

- 'Walks up *stairs* both feet together on each stair' was modified to read:
  'Walks up *steps* both feet together on each step.'
- 'Helps himself/herself to reasonable spoonfuls' - was modified to read:
  'Helps himself/herself to reasonable mouthfuls.'
- 'Unbuttons accessible clothing' -was modified to read:
  'Unties/removes/unbuttons accessible clothing.'
- 'Can recognize coins up to 10p' - was modified to read:
  'Can recognize coins up to 25 cents.'

One problem facing the students was to reduce the number of skills to a manageable size. An attempt was made to overcome this problem when the four groups had completed their work and they were brought together for discussions of the proposed assessment chart.

The total number of skills suggested by the students was 188. However, as a result of much discussion, the total number was reduced to 165. An attempt was made to produce an assessment chart that was not too unwieldy and yet was as comprehensive as possible. The Basic Assessment Chart still contained a substantial number of skills and, with hindsight, probably three or four skills could have been added to Occupational Skills under sub-area 'agility', e.g. 'Is able to jump using both feet'; 'Is able to throw an object and hit a target 4 to 5 feet away'; 'Uses large school apparatus in a safe manner'. After all, gross motor skills are particularly important in a predominantly rural economy. The author was accepted as the final arbitrator and he decided to merge certain skills to form one major skill. For example, 'Brushes hair (boys)' and 'Combs hair (girls)' were replaced by 'Able to wash hair adequately'. It was agreed that this skill is regarded in Sri Lanka as more important than the other two skills. During the discussion, reference was made to life-skills objectives relevant to the design of learning systems both in the in-school and out-of-school situation. It was within a framework of life-skills of objectives that the skills were agreed upon.

The students provided several sub-skills for one major skill, and, even though this was gratifying because it reflected the emphasis which had been placed on the breaking down of skills into sub-skills (task analysis), for the purpose of the Basic Assessment Chart many sub-skills had to be removed. For example, the following 13 sub-skills were replaced by 8 skills (See Appendix, Self-help Skills, 1-8):

- will take liquid from a cup when held to lips;
- takes solids well;
- puts hands around cup when drinking;
- holds, bites and chews;
- feeds self with fingers;
- drinks from cup with assistance;
- feeds self but spills a lot;
- manages a cup well without spilling;
- feeds self, only occasionally spilling;
- feeds himself/herself fairly well;
- can drink from ordinary mug which is almost full, without spilling;
- eats quite skilfully;
- pours water from one mug to another.

The content of the Basic Assessment Chart was divided into 13 sub-areas (Table 1). (It is appreciated that many skills will not be mastered by some young mentally retarded children, but one would expect a progression in mastery as the children grow older). Each group of students provided an English and a Sinhala version of their respective area of study. The students were continually reminded that the construction of the Basic Assessment Chart was expeimental and open-ended. They were encouraged to give even further thought to the exercise which they had completed and to be prepared to modify the chart as they thought necessary, but to remember to refer to authorities of the subject.

It is hoped that the results of future work in this field will be used in conjunction with a standardized test of intelligence when this has been developed in Sri Lanka. It must be emphasized at this juncture, that virtually nothing had been developed in the area of developmental assessment, not only for mentally retarded but for all children.

Table 1. Content of the Basic Assessment Chart

Skill Area	No. of Items
SELF-HELP SKILLS:	
Eating habits	10
Mobility	14
Toilet and washing	10
Dressing	10
COMMUNICATION SKILLS:	
Language	13
Differences	12
Number and money	22
Time and measure	8
Reading and writing	17
SOCIALIZATION SKILLS:	
Play activities and social relationships	16
Home activities and shopping	19
OCCUPATIONAL SKILLS:	
Dexterity	10
Agility	4

It was stressed that even though one would encounter older, severely mentally retarded children who would have many gaps in their social competence, according to the results of the Basic Assessment Chart, more systematic teaching would help these children achieve certain skills sooner and more effectively than previously thought. This point was quite deliberately stressed in an attempt to make teachers of these children more ambitious. It is possible that with these children certain skills may only be acquired in adulthood, but it may well be that these skills could be acquired in childhood provided that teachers are made aware of the importance of the skills and the need to teach them. Furthermore,it may well be found that for some children some of the skills are too 'adult' and need to be replaced by easier ones (and vice versa), but this is where the students should use their ingenuity and continually modify and innovate.

However, it was stressed that even certain social maturity scales devised for the pre-school level are frequently too high for the severely and profoundly retarded and/or have too large a gap between skills to accurately assess the level of functioning of many of these children. This means that, due to the infantile functioning level of some of these children and the small achievement increments made over time, it is imperative that teachers of the severely and profoundly retarded have a thorough working knowledge of human growth and development patterns from birth to pre-shcool, as well as the basic readiness and early academic learning processes. A high degree of insight into child development during the infancy stage, such as visual tracking, responding to stimuli, lifting the head, reaching for objects, and turning over is needed since it is within this range of functioning that teachers will find many of the severely and profoundly retarded. In this respect the PIP Developmental Charts (Jeffree & McConkey, 1976) were invaluable These charts contain a list of skills that children learn during the early months and years of life.

TASK ANALYTIC PROCEDURES

The use of the Basic Assessment Chart led to a discussion of the use of task analytic procedures. The students were shown how task analysis may be regarded as an effective method for teaching skills to handicapped individuals. Demonstrations were used in the homes/schools to show how a target skill can be analyzed into its component behaviors. It was demonstrated how each component behavior is learned sequentially and separately and is chained to those behaviors previously learned, until the complete task can be performed without assistance. Task analytic procedures for assessment and evaluation were demonstrated by adopting the same approach.

The use of task analytic procedures led to the refining of the information obtained from the use of the Basic Assessment Chart which contained items or 'priority behaviors'. These 'priority behaviors' were selected because they were regarded as essential stages in the development of the target skill being assessed. Furthermore, these procedures provided a format which was extremely useful in developing teaching programs. When these items were carefully selected, they provided a ready-made set of teaching objectives. A curriculum which has clear objectives in terms of specified skills will permit careful assessment of each child's abilities and will enable selection of an appropriate item as the next teaching target for that individual. It will provide a structure by means of which the person is able to progress, by small steps, through a hierarchy of skills, which is not based on normative developmental data, but on the breakdown of target skills into constituent elements by a process of task analysis.

The author emphasized that assessment procedure must be relevant to a teaching program and it must ensure that the skills being measured are appropriate to the degree of handicap. Therefore, the assessment must be composed of functional, practical items which measure many broad areas of function.

CONCLUSIONS

The design of the Basic Assessment Chart was an integral part of the discussion of a curriculum for the mentally retarded, using a behavioral objectives approach. It had been decided that there are areas of a curriculum that are common to most children. In other words, a discussion of a 'core' curriculum took place along the lines of Crawford (1980) and Gardner et. al. (1983). A summary of the model used is as follows:

- identify the 'core' areas of the curriculum;
- sub-divide these 'core' areas into their component parts;
- write targets for each component;
- device a standard assessment for competence in relation to the targets;
- use task analysis to break down each target into a hierarchy of skills and prepare a program to teach the target skills; and
- devise a record-keeping system.

It was extremely difficult to select the 165 skills mainly because the students were so enthusiastic and ambitious. However, much benefit was derived from these difficulties because the students were appreciating the sub-skills which had to be mastered before a target skill could be achieved.

The exercise was also extremely rewarding in that the chart was completed by students who would eventually be teaching mentally retarded children and serving as 'pioneers' in the field of mental retardation. It was particularly rewarding to observe the tremendous amount of effort and conscientiousness being put into the task. The debate concerning the composition of the chart continued until the end of the one-year course, and, particularly, when the students were completing their child studies. Obviously, there were many skills which should have been included but did not find a place. Several students were already discussing the possibility of devising additional charts. Copies of the Basic Assessment Chart were presented to the class teachers at the homes/schools, and the Sinhala version was particularly beneficial to the non-English speaking staff and aides.

No attempt was made to provide a mental or social age. The chart is not normative, but it does provide a substantial list of skills which the teacher can use to assess the child and note his capacities, his weaknesses, as well as the likely 'next skills' to concentrate on within each area. The chart measures a person's attainment on a particular functional, practical skill which, if taught, would allow him/her to exercise and extend his/her degree of independence. This assessment, together with task analytic procedures as a refinement, has obvious advantages over norm-referenced tests because of its relationship to the teaching program. Furthermore, many forms of assessment contain items which are arranged in order of difficulty and measure the same broad area of skill but individual items may have no direct relationship to the preceding items, other than being more difficult to achieve. In the case of the Basic Assessment Chart, task analytic procedures are an integral part of the whole assessment procedure.

The importance of the Basic Assessment Chart for teachers of the mentally retarded in Sri Lanka is that, in determining a child's level of development in certain 'core' areas and individual needs, it provides a baseline from which to plan for the next stage of his/her development. Initial assessment provides the child's entry point into a curriculum and should result in a 'written plan of development suited to his individual needs' (Mittler, 1979b). Furthermore, planning for development implies a periodic review of a child's progress and assessment needs.

References

Carr, J. (1982). *Helping your handicapped child.* London: Penguin.

CESA 12 (1975). *Portage project material. Portage: a guide to education.* Windsor: NFER/Nelson.

Crawford, N.B. (ed.)(1980). *Curriculum planning for the ESN(S) child.* Kiddnerminster: British Institute of Mental Handicap.

Gardner, J., Murphy, J. & Crawford, N.B. (1983). *The skills analysis model.* Kidderminster: British Institute of Mental Handicap.

Gunzburg, H.C. (1974). *Progress assessment charts.* Birmingham: SEFA (Publications) Ltd.

Hughes, J.M. (1977). *Helping the mentally retarded.* Colombo: Ceylon Association for the Mentally Retarded. (Sinhala version, 1980).

Hughes, J.M. (1981). The problem of identification of mental retardation in developing countries with special reference to Sri Lanka. *Teaching and Training, 19*(2) 39-46.

Jeffree, D.M. & McConkey, R. (1976). *PIP development charts.* London: Hodder & Stoughton.

Jeffree, D.M. Cheseldine, S. (1983). *Pathways to independence.* London: Hodder & Stoughton.

Kiernan, C. & Jones, M. (1977). *Behavior assessment battery.* Slough: NFER/Nelson.

Mittler, P. (1979a). Parents and teachers in special education. *Education for development.* (University College of Cardiff) 5(3) 19-27.

Mittler, P. (1979b). *People and patients.* London: Methuen.

Simon, G.B. (1981). *The next step on the ladder.* Kidderminster: British Institute of Mental Handicap.

Whelan, E. & Speake, B. (1979). *Learning to cope.* London: Souvenir Press.

APPENDIX

A BASIC ASSESSMENT CHART FOR USE WITH MENTALLY RETARDED CHILDREN IN SRI LANKA

Self-help Skills

Eating habits

Can feed him/herself without requiring assistance.
Can drink without spilling, holding container in one hand.
Is capable of helping him/herself to a drink.
Serves him/herself and eats without much assistance.
Can pour liquids.
Sits correctly to eat his/her meal.
Asks to have food passed to him/her.
Is able to help him/herself to reasonable mouthfuls.
Washes hands before meals without being told to do so.
Washes hands after meals.

Mobility

1. Can walk up steps with both feet together on each step.
2. Can walk down steps with both feet together on each step.
3. Uses a play vehicle of some kind.
4. Can walk up steps, one foot per step, without supporting him/herself.
5. Can walk down steps, one foot per step, without supporting him/herself.
6. Is able to go to neighbors and places nearby.
7. Requires little supervision playing outside home—absent for some time.
8. Wanders about without need for much supervision.
9. Wanders about neighborhood unsupervised, but does not cross main road.
10. Wanders about neighborhood unsupervised—crosses road.
11. Is able to walk across a room carrying a container of food and drinks without spilling.
12. Is able to get on and off trains and buses without difficulty.
13. Is able to go to correct side of road or platform for bus or train.
14. Recognizes and knows the meaning of traffic signals (mechanical and human)

Toilet and washing

1. Is toilet-trained and has few accidents.
2. Asks to go to toilet or is able to go him/herself.
3. Is able to care for him/herself at toilet and cleans him/herself.
4. Washes and cleans his/her hands in an acceptable way.
5. Is able to wash face more or less adequately.
6. Washes him/herself adequately and completely without much supervision.
7. Is able to prepare everything for washing him/herself.
8. Is able to wash hair adequately.
9. Keeps hands and face adequately clean without having to be told.
10. Changes clothes if soiled.

Dressing

1. Assists when he/she is being dressed.
2. Is able to remove and put on simple articles of clothing.
3. Unties/removes/unbuttons accessible clothing.
4. Undresses at night with little assistance.
5. Dresses in the morning with little assistance.
6. Is able to put on most ordinary clothes.
7. Is able to dress him/herself in a tidy fashion.
8. Takes responsible care of clothes and avoids soiling them excessively.
9. Takes reasonable care of clothes when undressing, folds them, puts them away, etc.

Communication

Language

1. Obeys simple instructions.
2. Understands orders containing: on, in, behind, under, above, in front of, underneath.
3. Is able to relate experiences in a coherent way.
4. Uses sentences containing plurals, past tense, prepositions.
5. Comprehends simple questions and gives sensible answers.
6. Is able to define simple words.
7. Can use involved sentences containing: because, but, etc.
8. Is able to carry out a 'triple order', e.g. put this... the... and then ....
9. Understands directions: top left, bottom right, etc.
10. Repeats a short story without much difficulty.
11. Is able to give his/her full name and address when asked to do so.
12. Is able to give age and birthday.

13. Understands words relating to quantities.

Differences

1. Is able to appreciate sex differences, e.g. man, woman, boy, girl.
2. Is able to discriminate colors by matching.
3. Differentiates between short, long; big, small; thick, thin.
4. Discriminates and names four or more colors without making a mistake.
5. Is able to refer correctly to 'morning' and 'afternoon'.
6. Is able to appreciate 'left' and 'right' on him/herself e.g. left arm, right ear
7. Is able to name days of the week, and recognizes some days in print.
8. Understands difference between: day-week, minute-hour, etc.
9. Differentiates between heavy and light, high and low, above and below, on and off, full and empty.
10. Understands sizes—large, medium and small.
11. Discriminates between shades of colour and understands adjectives pale, dark, bright, light.
12. Is able to follow directions involving left and right.

Number and money

1. Is able to differentiate between one thing and many things.
2. Understands the difference between two and many things.
3. Is able to count mechanically ten objects.
4. Is able to understand number situations up to four (including subtraction).
5. Is able to arrange objects in order of size from the smallest to the largest.
6. Is able to count mechanically twenty or more objects.
7. Is able to understand number situations up to 13 or more (including subtraction).
8. Is able to recognize coins up to 25 cents.
9. Is able to add coins of various denominations up to 25 cents.
10. Is able to give change/balance up to 25 cents.
11. Is able to count correctly up to 40 objects (e.g. coins).
12. Is able to say without much difficulty whether coins of various denominations are more or less than others.
13. Is able to give the figure before and after a given example without having to start counting again, e.g. 8 is before 9, 10 is after 9.
14. Is able to count correctly up to 70 objects.
15. Is able to count mechanically by 10s up to 60.

16. Follows instructions: Turn to page... (number under 100).
17. Is able to count mechanically by 5s up to 40.
18. When given various coins, can make up amounts to 25 cents.
19. When given various coins, can make up amounts to 50 cents.
20. Associates printed prices up to one Rupee with correct amount of money.
21. Associates printed prices up to two Rupees with correct amount of money,
22. Associates printed prices up to five Rupees with correct amount of money.

Time and measure

1. Knows how many days in a week.
2. Is able to name days of the week in order.
3. Is able to say what day it will be tomorrow.
4. Knows which day of the week it is and gives correct month and year.
5. Understands concepts of half and quarter with clock.
6. Is able to use a measuring container to measure one pint, one and a half pints, one cup, half cup.
7. Assosciates printed time with correct time on the clock.
8. Is able to use a scale for telling weight, e.g. can weigh 'parcels' of various sizes.

Reading and writing

1. Holds pencil or crayon and can imitate vertical and circular strokes.
2. Is able to copy circles.
3. Is able to draw a primitive man showing head and legs.
4. Is able to draw recognizable 'men' and huts/houses.
5. Is able to print his/her name and recognize it among other printed words and names.
6. Is able to recognize 25 words or more words of everyday usage.
7. Is able to read simple instructions, e.g. on public transport.
8. Is able to write own address.
9. Is able to read simple reading matter.
10. Recognizes his/her own name and those of at least three of his/her peers.
11. Is able to read food labels.
12. Makes a 'shopping list' for his/her own use.
13. Is able to read and write numbers in figures up to 100 (no reversals).

14. Is able to read simple messages printed for him, and understands them.
15. Writes simple sentences.
16. Is able to read books suitable for six-year-olds.
17. Is able to read books suitable for nine-year-olds.

Socialization

Play activities and social relationships

1. Plays in company with others, but does not yet co-operate with others.
2. Waits his/her turn, can 'share' with others, at times.
3. Plays cooperatively with others.
4. Enjoys entertaining others.
5. Is involved in competitive games, e.g. hide and seek.
6. Acts out stories he/she has heard.
7. Sings and/or dances to music.
8. Plays simple ball games with others.
9. Plays cooperative team games.
10. Is able to give the full names of at least 6 different people in his/her peer group.
11. Is able to refer to at least 6 different people by name (not immediate family or peers), recognizes them and addresses them correctly.
12. Is able to differentiate between his/her own relatives, e.g. refers correctly to his/her own aunt, cousin, etc.
13. Takes reasonable care of things which belong to other people.
14. Is able to ask for help or information from friends, teachers, etc.
15. Is quite well-behaved outside his/her own home, e.g. other people's homes.
16. Asks for help or information from strangers.

Home activities and shopping

1. Fetches and carries on request.
2. Shows that he/she can help in domestic tasks, e.g. cleaning table, sweeping, etc.
3. Is able to go on simple errands outside the home.
4. Is able to go to shops while adult waits outside.
5. Is trusted with money while on errands.
6. Is able to go to one shop and purchase specified items.
7. Is able to take on minor responsiblities.
8. Is able to go to several shops or stores to fetch specified items.

9. Carries out minor routine tasks without supervision, e.g. fetching water.
10. Is able to do simple tasks without supervision.
11. Prepares dishes for washing (i.e. removes scraps from dishes) and washes them satisfactorily.
12. Is able to clean up any mess caused accidentally.
13. Is able to tidy/make his/her own bed in the morning.
14. Tidies up after his/her own activities without having to be asked.
15. Finds the appropriate shop or stall for buying simple items.
16. Is able to choose the item he/she wants from a selection.
17. Shows that he/she has a realistic idea of some everyday prices.
18. Is able to hand over the correct money when buying an item.
19. Has at least an approximate idea of prices of some common foods.

Occupation

Dexterity (Fine finger movements)

1. Is able to string large beads.
2. Is able to unscrew lids with a twisting movement.
3. Cuts paper with scissors.
4. Is able to make constructive use of clay, blocks, etc.
5. Cuts out pictures with scissors.
6. Is able to wind thread fairly evenly onto a spool.
7. Is able to cut cloth with scissors.
8. Is able to pile papers, cards, etc. in a neat way.
9. Cuts very accurately around outlines.
10. Is able to make an acceptable parcel using paper and cord.

Agility (Gross motor control)

1. Is able to kick ball/box without falling.
2. Is able to stand tip-toe for 10 seconds.
3. Uses hammer and nails to put two pieces of wood together.
4. Uses garden/farm and kitchen tools.

11

EDUCATIONAL SERVICES FOR THE MENTALLY RETARDED IN DEVELOPING COUNTRIES

John M. Hughes

FACTORS AFFECTING EDUCATIONAL GROWTH IN DEVELOPING COUNTRIES

There is an abundance of evidence to suggest that many developing countries are rapidly approaching their budgetary ceilings for educational expenditure and, at the same time, are failing to reach their educational targets (UNESCO, 1975a; Thomas, 1975; Smith, 1979; O'Leary, 1980). Obviously, it is essential that any study and discussion concerning the provision of educational services for the mentally retarded in developing countries must take place within the context of existing educational systems and the problems of educational growth in these countries. Furthermore, these educational services must be considered as realistically as possible within the limited resources of the country concerned. The high levels of drop-out and repetition of grades being experienced by many developing countries must surely be a serious obstacle to the attainment of national development goals such as universal primary education, eradication of illiteracy and equality of educational opportunity (Abraham, 1982; UNESCO, 1975b, 1979a).

Against this background of problems involved in the growth of educational services in developing countries, one finds the mentally retarded, who are the largest single group of those children who, through the possession of mental or physical handicaps, are at social and educational risk. The numbers are so significant that, even in countries with well-developed educational systems, they create serious problems for the allocation of resources. In those countries which are still in the process of developing their educational systems, these persons raise the issue of social and financial priority because the vast majority can, given adequate support and services, live productive and fulfilled lives.

ASSESSING THE EXTENT OF THE PROBLEM OF MENTAL RETARDATION IN DEVELOPING COUNTRIES

As in the pre-industrialized society of the U.K., so in the rural communities of developing countries varying degrees of mental retardation can easily pass unnoticed because the degree of retardation does not inconvenience the 'affected' person and does not ostracize him from the social group. In other words, the person may not be regarded as 'mentally retarded' or unusual in some way in the rural community because, even though his level of intellectual functioning (assuming one is able to measure his level) is well below average, in his own rural community, he is 'socially competent' and 'socially acceptable'. He merges imperceptibly with his fellow villagers and is able to cope quite well with the incidents and hazards that might arise in his lifetime.

This brings one to the conclusion that mental retardation is not really a thing in itself, but involves the way in which a particular society reacts to its less able citizens. In many developing countries, very few people are regarded as being mentally retarded; there may be few opportunities for schooling and most of the population may be occupied with unskilled work. However, in a highly developed country where most parents have greater expectations for their children, they may seek, expect and frequently demand special help for the less able.

As an individual's society develops technical sophistication, so the limited resources resulting from his intellectual handicap to his technical sophistication will begin to matter to him and to other members of his society. This means that, as development spreads to the more remote areas of a country, or when the individual moves to the industrializing towns and cities; the education, health and social services will have to accept more responsibility for the identification, diagnosis, assessment, education, rehabilitation and protection of this person. In 1950, there were only six cities in the world with a population of 5 million or more; by 1980, the figure had risen to 26 cities, and by the year 2000, there will probably be 60 such cities with a total of 650 million (Salas, 1980).

Information provided by international agencies (Commonwealth Secretariat, 1971; Hughes, 1983; UNESCO, 1979b, 1981a; WHO, 1968,

1975) reflects the difficulty involved in assessing the size of the prevalence of mental retardation in developing countries. Estimates of prevalence are not only affected by the fact that mentally retarded persons are more like other people than they are different, but are affected by public awareness of the existence of mental retardation, the limits and scope of investigations, and the definitions used. A further factor that influences the identification of mental retardation and other handicaps in developing countries is the influence of public attitudes and cultural practices (Hughes, 1983; Miles, 1983). As in many developed countries, fear and ignorance in developing countries combine to influence public and parental attitudes to the mentally retarded. This factor was highlighted by some parents of handicapped children in Sri Lanka who hid their children from sight because of embarrassment which arose from personal or religious and superstitious reasons, or because the members of the community believed that the handicap was contagious (Hughes, 1980a; 1982a,b; 1983).

Prevalence is influenced by complex interacting factors. High infant mortality in many countries reduces the number of severe cases. However, as one looks to the future, one can anticipate a growing problem resulting from the increasing survival rates of severe cases as a result of the advancement of medical science, improving standards of living, and other improvements in developing countries. It appears that the development of a country tends to create greater problems of mental retardation. Many children in developing countries suffer from severe protein malnutrition (PEM). There is evidence which suggests that malnutrition may work directly on the developing brain; it may work by increasing the child's vulnerability to infectious disease; or it may work by diminishing responsiveness and hence opportunity for learning, for prolonged periods of time (Hughes, 1980a; Perkins, 1979; Reed, 1979; Righter, 1980).

THE PROBLEMS OF IDENTIFICATION AND ASSESSMENT OF MENTAL RETARDATION

The elaborate screening systems being devised in the richer developed countries of the world will take many years to be developed in the Third World. No real attempt has been made in most of these countries to identify children suffering from mental retardation (UNESCO, 1979b). Kysela and Marfo (1984) provide a model for screening and intervention procedures based on the health care system of Ghana. Omari and Kisanji (1984) provide a similar model for Tanzania, and child care staff are being trained in this area in

Jamaica (Thorburn, 1984).

However, it is possible that basic screening procedures can arise as a result of the efforts being made, in many developing countries, to ensure that as many as possible of the population are moved out of the poverty band and that they receive advice on nutrition and primary health care. The identification of children requiring special educational treatment could arise from the development of primary health schemes and the organization of para-medical teams along the lines of the 'bare-foot' doctors of China (Hughes, 1981; 1983). Obviously, much of their work would involve advice on nutrition, basic hygiene, general primary health care and basic medical treatment. These teams could contribute to the provision of educational services by accumulating data on the incidence and distribution of various forms of handicap. However, there is one very important factor to consider if one intends to consider educational services for mentally retarded and other handicapped children. One must be realistic and fully appreciate the prevailing social and economic conditions of the country concerned. This means that, even though these children are identified, it does not mean that, if they are enrolled at school, they will receive appropriate education—their teachers may lack sympathy and understanding of their problems. Furthermore, even when these children are identified, and when there are sympathetic and knowledgeable teachers waiting to teach them, the children may not attend school because of economic reasons. This last factor, more than any other, highlights the enormous task facing developing countries that wish to provide some form of educational service for these children.

Assessment: Assessment of the mentally retarded child implies an evaluation of the nature and extent of his intellectual, emotional, social, motor, and sensory assets and deficits. However, in most developing countries, there is a dearth of psychometric instruments and developmental scales (UNESCO, 1979b). These countries can benefit from the change in approach to assessment which has occurred in the Western World. This change of approach involves the growing awareness of the need to develop forms of assessment alternative to the standardized and conventional psychological tests. Basic to these alternative approaches is the concept of criterion-referenced measurement (Jeffree and McConkey, 1976; Jeffree, 1979; Whelan and Speake, 1980; Carr, 1980; Simon, 1981).

One very important conclusion arising from this change of approach, which is particularly applicable to developing countries, is the importance attached to the contribution that teachers can make to the comprehensive assessment of children. Furthermore, because of a dearth of psyschometric instruments, developmental scales will be the only means of assessing the child in many developing countries for some time to come. The responsibility for administering these assessment procedures is likely to fall upon the shoulders of teachers for some years, rather than educational psychologists. Therefore, there is an obvious need for teachers to receive guidance in the design and use of basic assessment scales along the lines of those developed by the author in Sri Lanka (Chapter 10 of this volume; see also Hughes, 1977, 1980, 1983); Miles (1980) in Pakistan; Kysela and Marfo (1984) in Ghana; Zaman and Akhtar (1984) in Bangladesh and the WHO Community Rehabilitation Manual. In this way, teachers will begin to appreciate the use and the importance of task analytic procedures and prepare the way for educational programs that will meet the needs of individual children.

THE ORGANIZATION OF EDUCTIONAL SERVICES FOR THE MENTALLY RETARDED

Developing countries should have national policies in special education directed to the aims of providing equal access for all to education and the integration of all citizens into the economic and social life of the community. In this respect, special education should be regarded as a branch of general education.

Many governments in developing countries have accepted responsibility, in principle, for the care of handicapped children and young children in general but the realistic situation is that they are unable to allocate funds commensurate with the need. Present available evidence indicates that very few of these countries provide eduational services for the mentally retarded (Commonwealth Secretariat, 1977; UNESCO, 1981a). Even where educational services do exist, this provision is very meagre indeed and countries depend upon agencies other than the national government to supply initiative, personnel and finance for the care, education and rehabilitation of the mentally retarded. However, some countries do not yet have effective national associations which can provide facilities, influence a government on behalf of the mentally retarded, or encourage the development of national voluntary agencies to promote the education and welfare of the mentally retarded.

There is a need for governments to increase their assistance to voluntary agencies and encourage them to concentrate their resources on those children who are at a level characterized by the dominance of 'care problems' and the need for almost full time attention to self-help skills. Furthermore, use should be made of appropriately modified WHO Community Rehabilitation Schemes and the results of the current UNICEF programs in "Reaching the Unreached" in such countries as Zambia and Philippines.

Wherever possible, the mildly mentally retarded should be accommodated in the ordinary schools and educated as closely as possible to the mainstream of educational services in ordinary classes, taking into account their special needs and the needs of other children. In view of the virtual non-existence of special educational provision for the mentally retarded within many educational systems and the enormous cost of providing special schools compared to the relatively lower cost of integration, the maximum integration of the mildly retarded into ordinary schools and classes should take place.

It must be emphasized, however, that the establishment of a special class or the integration of children into the ordinary class is no guarantee of excellence. The need for courses of teacher training to contain a common core course on 'children with special educational needs' becomes imperative. The skill and knowledge of the teacher is vital in any form of educational service for these children. This exerts a more potent influence than any form of organization. However, those responsible for the education of the mentally retarded, and other handicapped children should study the findings and comments of special educators and agencies in various parts of the world on the subject of integration —those who offer warnings and cautions (Mba, 1977; Cruickshank, 1979; Hegarty and Pocklington, 1981) and those who offer more optimistic opinions and evalutions (Chazan and Laing, 1980; Guerin and Szatlocky, 1979; Hegarty and Pocklington, 1982; 1981; UNESCO, 1979b).

TEACHER TRAINING FACILITIES IN SPECIAL EDUCATION

When it is appreciated that at least 75% of mentally retarded children are mildly retarded, and that, even in developed countries (e.g. U.K.), the majority of these are found in ordinary schools (Kushlick and Blunden, 1974), then it becomes essential that all teacher training courses should contain a substantial special education element. The effectiveness of any kind of provision for these children will depend largely upon the skill, knowledge and enthusiasm of the teachers. However, present available evidence indicates that many teachers in developing countries are not professionally trained (Smith, 1979), and there are very few countries with training facilities for teachers of mentally retarded children, or for children exhibiting other learning difficulties (Commonwealth Secretariat, 1977; UNESCO, 1979b, 1981a). However one should give due credit to the attempts being made to develop staff training in, for example, the Caribbean, India, Philippines and Nepal.

The inclusion of a special education element covering 'children with special educational needs' is particularly relevant in developing countries because of the many adverse factors in the environment of the child. For example, poverty fosters many conditions, including overcrowding, poor standards of hygiene, ignorance and superstition, which in turn, nurture malnutrition and disease resulting in both physical and mental retardation. There should not only be a special education element in initial teacher training, but there should be a second stage of special education where a student has the opportunity to study the field in more depth. Such a person could then be regarded as a generalist—a person who is well-prepared for further study. This then, could be a start at providing a gradually increasing number of teachers who would be able to recognize children with various learning difficulties and provide intelligent and appropriate assistance (Friese, 1984).

However, there is an urgent need to train teacher educators in special education. In this respect, there is a need to provide developing countries with aid in the form of scholarship schemes so that teachers can study special education in other countries. The University of Wales is about to offer a B.Ed. option entitled 'Special Education for Developing Countries' (Hughes, in press).

THE ARGUMENT FOR EDUCATIONAL SERVICES FOR THE MENTALLY RETARDED

Many people would probably doubt the advisability of suggesting that money and resources should be spent on the handicapped in developing countries because of the problems facing governments in their attempts to provide educational services for non-handicapped children. It can be appreciated that where governments are confronted by growing problems of unemployed school leavers, they may consider that developments in provision for the handicapped must be delayed until a future date when the situation might be more favorable. For example, in Bangladesh the people are still fighting to overcome the common enemies of poverty, disease, illiteracy, unemployment and rapid population growth. In this country, where over 80% are illiterate (UNESCO, 1979b), the provision of universal primary education is at present impossible.

In developing countries, the inclusion of the handicapped into the State system can only be considered if a sound, convincing argument can be put forward. In other words, educational services for the handicapped should be considered as something necessary for the handicapped and his family, not purely on humanitarian grounds, but also as something that will benefit the State. The argument advanced should state the economic advantage of providing resources during the early years rather than providing larger sums of money when the individual reaches adulthood. Much evidence is available in developed countries to suggest that money spent on the handicapped provides a good return for investment. However, one must ask the question whether this evidence is applicable to the reality of the Third World. For example, this particular evidence places emphasis on the investment in 'rehabilitation' and 'vocational' training rather than on special education during the early years of the individual; on the saving of money as a result of not providing institutional care and social security benefits; and on the return of money to the government in the form of taxes (Conley, 1973; UNESCO, 1978). However, there are very few institutions for these people in developing countries and very few of these countries provide social security benefits.

What is particularly relevant to the situation in developing countries is that the major benefit derived from improved education and training of the mentally retarded is the increased independence and ability to perform daily tasks, particularly with the more severe cases. This has the practical result that the person becomes more self-competent and may be able to live (and work) in the community. As well as enabling him or her to live a more normal life, this will have practical benefits in terms of reduced 'cost' to the community. Furthermore, the argument should be based on 'earnings foregone'. This means that the handicapped frequently cost members of their family, or community, money in terms of earnings lost while the handicapped person is cared for or supervised.

The education of mentally retarded and other handicapped persons is a necessary component of a comprehensive human development service system. If there is an absence of eduational services for these persons, many are likely to suffer a degree of social incompetence and inadequacy and live well below the level of their potential.

In conclusion, I would wish to stress that those of us who are concerned for the right of handicapped persons to a life with some degree of human worth and dignity, must consider what realistic assistance we can provide to these people in order to enable them to survive, to help themselves, and to achieve worthwhile goals.

References

Abraham, A. S. (1982). Bid to curb drop-out rate. *Times Educational Supplement,* 7 May, p.7.

Barros, F. M. (1979). Cradled in hunger. *UNESCO Courier* January, 9-12.

Carr, J. (1980). *Helping your handicapped child.* London: Penguin.

Chazan, M. & Laing, A. (1980). *Some of our children: The education and care of young children with special needs.* London: Open Books.

Commonwealth Secretariat. (1971). *Directory of special educational provision for handicapped children in developing Commonwealth countries.* London: Commonwealth Secretariat.

Commonwealth Secretariat. (1977). *Education and training resources in the developing countries of the Commonwealth.* London: Commonwealth Secretariat.

Conley, R. (1973). *The economics of mental retardation.* Baltimore: The Johns Hopkins Press.

Cruickshank, W. M. (1979). Myths and realities in learning disabilities. In A. Lane (Ed.), *Readings in human growth and development of the exceptional individual* (pp. 58-64). Basingstoke: Globe Education.

Friese, A. J. (1984). *Perspectives of mental retardation in a Third World country: Implications for teacher education.* Paper presented at the 6th Congress of the International Association for the Scientific Study of Mental Deficiency, Toronto, Canada.

Guerin, F. R & Szatlocky, K. (1979). Integration programs for the mildly retarded. In *Readings in mental retardation.* (pp.108-113). Basingstoke: Globe Education.

Hegarty, S. & Pocklington, K. (1981). *Educating pupils with special needs in the ordinary school.* Slough: NFER/Nelson.

Hegarty, S. & Pocklington, K. (1982). *Integration in Action.* Slough: NFER/Nelson.

Hughes, J. M. (1977). *Helping the mentally retarded.* (Sinhala version, 1980). Colombo: Ceylon Association for the Mentally Retarded.

Hughes, J. M. (1980a). Malnutrition and mental retardation in developing countries. *Teaching and Training, 18*(1), 3-8.

Hughes, J. M. (1980b). Supem Uyana—the Garden of Love. *Teaching and Training, 18*(1), 25-29.

Hughes J. M. (1981). The problem of identification of mental retardation in developing countries with special reference to Sri Lanka. *Teaching and Training, 19*(2), 39-46.

Hughes, J. M. (1982a). Mental retardation in Sri Lanka and the influence of astrology. *Teaching and Training, 20*(1), 23-27.

Hughes, J. M. (1982b). *Educational services for the mentally retarded in developing countries.* Paper presented at the 6th Congress of the International Association for the Scientific Study of Mental Deficiency, Toronto, Canada.

Hughes, J. M. (1983). The mentally retarded in developing Commonwealth countries. *Education for Development* (University College, Cardiff), *June,* 11-19.

Hughes, J. M. (In press). Special education courses for Third World students: The influence of tradition, social complexity and cultural philosophy. *Education for Development.*

Jeffree, D. M. & McConkey, R. (1976). *PIP Developmental Charts.* London: Hodder and Stoughton.

Jeffree, D. M. (1979). *Pathways to independence.* London: Heodder and Stoughton.

Kushlick, A. & Blunden, R. (1974); The epidemiology of mental subnormality. In A. M. Clarke & A. D. B. Clarke (Eds.). *Mental deficiency: The changing outlook* (pp. 32-33). London: Methuen.

Kysela, G.M. & Marfo, K. (1984). Early handicapping conditions: detection and intervention in developing contries. In J. Berg (Ed.). *Perspectives and progress in mental retardation: Vol. I. Social, psychological, and educational aspects.* (pp. 119-130). Baltimore: University Park Press.

Mba, P. O. (1977). Special education in regular teacher education: some implications. Lagos: Nigerian Educational Research Council.

Miles, M. (1980). A school on the North West Frontier. *Special Education: Forward Trends, 7*(2), 32-33

Miles, M. (1983). *Attitudes towards persons with disabilities.* Peshawar: Mental Health Center, Mission Hospital.

O'Leary, J. (1980). Costs keep primary goals out of reach. *Times Educational Supplement, 22* August, p.11.

Omari, I. M. & Kisanji, J. A. N. (1984). *Screening and intervention with young retarded children in East Africa.* Paper presented at the 6th Congress of the International Association for the Scientific Study of Mental Deficiency, Toronto, Canada.

Perkins, S. A. (1979). Malnutrition and mental development. In A. Lane (Ed.). *Readings in human growth and development of the exceptional individual* (pp. 70-74). Baingstoke: Globe Education.

Reed, H. B. C. (1979). Biological defects and special education: an issue in personal preparation. *Journal of Special Education, 13*(1), 9-33.

Righter, R. (1980). The Eighties: Now the apocalypse? *Sunday Times,* 6 January, p.12.

Salas, R. M. (1980). *International population assistance—the first decade.* Oxford: Pergamon Press.

Simon, G. B. (1981). *The next step on the ladder.* Kidderminster: The British Institute for Mental Handicap.

Smith, R. L. (1979). *Progress towards universal primary education.* London: Commonwealth Secretariat.

Thomas, J. (1975). *World problems in education: A brief analytic survey.* Paris: UNESCO.

Thorburn, J. M. (1984). *Training of child care staff in early detection and intervention.* Paper presented at the 6th Congress of the International Association for the Scientific Study o Mental Deficiency, Toronto, Canada.

UNESCO (1975a). *Population and school enrolment: A statistical analysis.* Paris: UNESCO.

UNESCO (1975b). *Wastage in primary education in Africa.* Paris: UNESCO.

UNESCO (1978). *Economic aspects of special education.* (p.16). Paris: UNESCO.

UNESCO (1979a). *Wastage in primary education: A statistical study of trends and patterns in repetition and drop-out.* Paris: UNESCO.

UNESCO (1979b). *Regional seminar on the education of mentally retarded children held at Macquarie University.* Paris: UNESCO.

UNESCO (1979c). *UNESCO expert meeting on special education.* Paris: UNESCO.

UNESCO (1981a). UNESCO statistics on special education. Paris: UNESCO.

UNESCO (1981b). *Handicapped children: early detection, intervention and education.* Paris: UNESCO.

Whelan, E. & Speake, B. (1980). *Learning to cope.* London: Souvenir Press.

WHO (1968). *Organization of services for the mentally retarded.* Geneva: WHO.

WHO (1975). WHO policy and program for disability, prevention and rehabilitation. Geneva: WHO.

WHO (1980). *Mental retardation: Prevention, amelioration and service delivery.* Geneva: WHO.

Zaman, S. S. & Akhtar, S. (1984). *Effects of early and late intervention among retarded children: Bangladesh experience.* Papere presented at the 6th Congress of the International Association for the Scientific Study of Mental Deficiency, Toronto, Canada.

12

THE CARE AND EDUCATION OF DISABLED CHILDREN IN BANGLADESH

Sultana S. Zaman

Bangladesh was established as a sovereign state on December 16, 1971. The area of the country is 143,998 square kilometers. According to the census report of March 1981, the country's population stood at 90 million of which 87% live in rural areas and 13% in the urban areas. Per capita income is approximately 100 U.S. dollars per year. It is one of the most densely populated areas of the world. The population of children in the country is more than 40 million, 46.7% of whom are below 14 years of age (Islam, 1984).

According to a *Statistical Yearbook of Bangladesh* report released in 1982, infant mortality in the country is 111.5 per 1,000 live births (110.4/1,000 male and 109.5/1,000 female). The death rate among children from 1 to 4 years is 34.3 per 1,000 live births. Diarrhea, malnutrition, poliomyelitis, pneumonia, whooping cough, and meningitis are the major causes of mortality and morbidity in children. The 1975-76 National Nutrition Survey of Rural Bangladesh indicated that 78.8% of children suffered from second or third degree malnutrition. Illiteracy, ignorance, lack of sanitation, and poverty play a major role in the evolution of malnutrition. With such a depressing picture of children in general, it is not surprising that the situation of disabled children in Bangladesh is worse. They are the worst sufferers, and the most neglected and uncared for among the children population in the country.

THE DEVELOPMENT OF SERVICES FOR THE HANDICAPPED

The government of Bangladesh, through the Social Welfare Department, initiated its activities of treatment, training, education, and rehabilitation of the physically handicapped in 1961. As a result, during the middle of 1962, four schools for the blind and the deaf were started in four Divisions of Bangladesh. This program has gradually expanded. In 1969, integrated special education classes for the blind and the deaf in regular schools were started on an experimental basis. A Vocational Training and Employment Rehabilitation Center for blind and deaf adults was established in 1979.

The Bangladesh Child Welfare Council, a voluntary agency, started the Crippled Children's Center in Dhaka in 1961. The aim of the Center since its inception has been to provide physiotherapy for physically handicapped children. Its programs have been expanded lately to a 50-bed hospital with the provision of an operation theater as well. In 1975, under the auspices of the Women's Voluntary Association (WVA), a residential home was established for crippled children from outside Dhaka who were undergoing treatment at the Rehabilitation Institute and Hospital for the Disabled. Cheshire Home which caters for physically handicapped children and adults started its residential home in 1975.

The Bangladesh National Society for the Blind (BNSB), a voluntary organization, was established in 1972. BNSB has taken up several programs for the prevention, treatment, training, and rehabilitation of blind persons in the country. In 1976, in collaboration with a West German voluntry organization, the Christoffel Blinden Mission, a vocation training center for the blind was started by BNSB in Dhaka City. Assistance for Blind Children (ABC) is of recent origin, dating from April 1978. Its function has been to help and aid blind children through BNSB and government aided schools.

The Bangladesh National Federation for the Blind has several programs for the education and training of the blind and has many branches all over the country. There is also the Bangladesh National Federation for the Deaf. Established in 1976, this organization has a school for the deaf in Dhaka City; this school has expanded considerably over the past few years. Several other voluntary organizations run a few more schools for the deaf in a number of districts.

In 1977, a voluntary organization named the Society for the Care and Education of Mentally Retarded Children (SCEMRC) was established. Mainly a parents's association, SCEMRC initially started with integrated special education classes for mentally retarded children in regular schools. In 1982 SCEMRC, in collaboration with the Norwegian Association for the Mentally Retarded (also a parents' organization), started a vocational training center and sheltered workshop for the adult retarded. This center has come to be known as the Bangladesh Institute for the Mentally Retarded (BIMR). Finally, in May 1984 the Bangladesh Protibondhi Foundation, a voluntary organization for developmentally disabled children, was born with the setting up of a school (named 'Kalyani') for mentally retarded children.

From the above discussion we can see that through government and nongovernment efforts, some work has been done for the disabled in Bangladesh. However, one of the main problems in planning for the education and rehabilitation of the physically and mentally handicapped has been the lack of data. No census report contains adequate data on the incidence of handicaps in this country.

INCIDENCE AND PREVALENCE OF MAJOR DISABILITIES

Although no systematic epidemiological studies on disability have been done in Bangladesh, some survey attempts and statistical data do exist in some areas of disability. In the sections which follow the few studies into specific disabilities will be summarized.

The Disabled Children in Dhaka Survey

A survey of disabled children in Dhaka City (Sobhan & Rahman, 1963) conducted jointly by a nongovernmental organization, the East Pakistan Child Welfare Council (now known as the Bangladesh Child Welfare Council) and the College of Social Welfare and Research in 1961 was a pioneer effort. The main purpose of the study was to collect statistical data on disabled children in Dhaka City in order to start work on the East Pakistan Child Welfare Council's Crippled Children's center (this center has expanded considerably).

The target of the survey was to cover one-fifth of the total population of Dhaka City. The total number of households and the population covered were 9,886 and 80,295 respectively. The greater part of the area covered fell in three old city and slum areas. A total of 245 disabled children were found in 229 families from among the whole population covered by the study. The major disabilities, according to this survey, were those involving the limbs (40.4%), hearing and speech (16.5%), and sight (15%). Most of the disabled children identified were in the 2- to 16-year age range (88.4%). Children below age 2 and those above 17 represented 3.2% and 8.4% of the population respectively.

Physically Handicapped Children in Bangladesh Study

A study of the situation of handicapped children in Bangladesh was conducted by the Institute of Social Welfare and Research, the University of Dhaka, and UNICEF in 1979 during the International Year of the Child (Mia, Islam, & Ali, 1979). The purpose of the study was to obtain baseline data for developing policies and programs to improve the opportunities available to the handicapped in private and public sectors. Dr. Michael Irwin, the then UNICEF representative in Bangladesh took keen interest in initiating and funding the study.

The survey was conducted in 8 rural unions from 4 administrative divisions and 6 wards from urban municipalities representing different sizes of towns. In the selected areas, all houses were enumerated for identification of handicapped children and then the households with handicapped children were interviewed for more detailed information. The results of the study indicated that the incidence rate of handicaps in children was 7.88 per 1,000 children below 15 years of age. The national child population in 1978 being 34.37 million, this rate gives a total of 285,460 handicapped children in the country of which 266,240 and 20,060 were rural and urban respectively.

If we compare the 1961 and 1979 studies, we do find considerable similarity in findings, although there are differences in sample selection and methodology. One striking similarity is that the organs most affected among the physically disabled are the legs, hands, and eyes. It could be that large numbers of children suffering from poliomyelitis, cerebral palsy, etc., have remained uncared for as services for these chidlren are meagre. Impairments of the eye have, however, received better attention not only by the government agencies but also by nongovernmental organizations.

International Epidemiological Studies of Childhood Disability

As part of the international epidemiological studies into childhood disability, a pilot study in Bangladesh was undertaken where a door to door survey of 1,005 children between ages 3 and 9 was conducted in 8 villages of Dhamrai Union of Dhaka District (Zaman, 1982). The total number of households visited was 590. Two questionnaires were administered to the mother while the children were observed to find out if they had any disabilities. Two hundred and fifteen children were identified through the questionnaires as having one or more disabling conditions. These children were then assessed in detail by a physician and a psychologist. The nature and degrees of disabilities

Table 1. Epidemiological Study of Childhood Disabilities: Breakdown of 215 Children Identified in Dhamrai Union

Condition	Number	%
Severe to moderate mental retardation	15	6.98
Mild mental retardation	126	58.60
Severe vision problem	16	7.44
Mild vision problem	22	10.23
Seizures	17	7.91
Hearing problem	8	3.72
Malnutrition	11	5.12
Total	215	100.00

found among these 3- to 9-year old children are summarized in Table 1.

Compared to the results from other developing countries where similar surveys have been conducted as part of the International Epidemiological Studies of Childhood Disability project, "children from Bangladesh are the most disadvantaged" is the comment by Dr. Lillian Belmont, the research scientist in charge of the study (see Belmont, 1984).

Case studies from the Child Guidance Clinic, Dhaka Medical College Hospital

Case histories of children who attended the Child Guidance Clinic of the Psychiatry Department of Dhaka Medical College Hospital from 1979 to 1982 were examined (Begum, 1983). A total of 295 children, the majority of them from middle class and poor families, attended the clinic during this period. The age group break-down is as follows: 120 children were between ages 11 and 15 years, 125 were between 6 and 10 years, while the remaining 50 children were below 5 years of age. The breakdown of the 295 children according to diagnostic categories was as follows:

- mental retardation—varying degrees (47.5%);
- speech problem (13.3%);
- neurotic problem (12.2%);

- psychotic problem (8.5%);
- epilepsy (8.5%);
- organic brain damage (5.1%); and
- Down's syndrome (5.1%).

Epidemiology of nutritional blindness: Xerophthalmia Prevalence Survey, 1982-83

Xerophthalmia is an eye disease caused by *vitamin A* deficiency. Blinding malnutrition in childhood is a serious public health problem in Bangladesh. The Bangladesh Program for the Prevention of Blindness, in collaboration with Helen Keller International supported a survey (conducted by the Institute of Health and Nutrition, Ministry of Health) to ascertain the prevalence of xerophthalmia among children below 6 years of age. The sample was taken from 82 sites representative of rural Bangladesh and 17 locations in slum areas of four major towns. A total of 11,624 rural and 2,271 urban households were visited to examine 18,660 rural and 3,675 urban children aged 3 months to 6 years. The results of this survey are summarized in Tables 2 and 3.

It was found also that 1,200 rural children under 6 years were among children with blindness from corneal destruction. At least 25,000 young children may be blinded each year, many failing to survive the acute blinding episode. About 45% (8 million) of rural children and 23% of children from urban slums had been given high potency *Vitamin A* capsules (VAC) through UNICEF. Corneal ulcers were almost three times more common in children not given VAC while night blindness rates were nearly double. The current target population receiving VAC is 18 million.

PROGRAMS FOR THE DISABLED IN BANGLADESH

Educational and training facilities for blind children

As has been stated earlier, xerophthalmia or nutritional blindness among children is a major public health problem in Bangladesh. It affects almost 5% of rural children under 6 years, about one million children overall. Once a child becomes blind, the services available to that child are meagre compared to the magnitude of the problem. However, some governmental as well as nongovernmental programs exist for these children.

Table 2. Distribution of Various Types of Xerophthalmis Among Rural Children and Overall Rates Per 1000

Xerophthalmia Type	Cases/18,600	Rate/1,000
Night blindness	674	35.7
Conjunctival Xerosis	362	19.5
Bitot spot	169	9.1
Corneal xerosis	10	0.5
Corneal ulceration	11	0.6
Corneal scar	39	2.5

Table 3. Distribution of Various Types of Xerophthalmia Among Urban Children and Overall Rates Per 1,000

Xerophthalmia Type	Cases/3,675	Rate/1,000
Night blindness	103	27.0
Conjunctival Xerosis	91	24.7
Bitot spot	58	15.8
Corneal xerosis	2	0.5
Corneal ulceration	2	0.5
Corneal scar	13	3.5

Government programs for the blind

Schools for the blind: The Department of Social Welfare runs 5 schools for blind children, one school, at least, in each of the four Divisions: Dhaka, Chittagong, Rajshahi, and Khulna. These schools have a total admission capacity of 500 children. The schools provide hostel facilities for a total of 160 children who receive free room and board at government expense. The rest of the students are day scholars. The schools provide formal education up to primary level class 5, and all students receive all instructional materials free of cost. Instruction is given in brialle and in such other areas as music and the vocational trades—mat making, weaving, cane chair production, etc.

Integrated education for blind children: The Department of Social Welfare has a scheme for the education of blind children with their sighted peers in 47 normal high schools all over the country. The scheme provides one resource teacher to each participating school and a resource room where the teacher works to help the blind students overcome their difficulties. The resource teacher also maintains contact with the families of the blind children to help deal with any problems they may have regarding the child's education. Under this scheme, a Braille Press donated by the American Foundation for Overseas Blind has been set up at Dhaka.

Training and rehabilitation of the adult blind: Four vocational training centers situated in four Divisional headquarters are attached to the four schools for the blind. Training in various trades are imparted by skilled instructors. A vocational training center and sheltered workshop has been set up for the adult blind in the industrial area of Tongi, Dhaka. This center is known as the Employment Rehabilitation Center and is supported by the International Labor Organization (ILO) and the Swedish International Development Agency (SIDA). A total of 150 blind persons receive training in this center. Training is offered in welding, fitting, light engineering work, plastic processing work, leather work, wood carving, and duck farming. At the end of the training many of the graduates are employed in nearby industries through the Placement Services section of the Center. Many of them go for higher training both at home and abroad. In 1981 one student from this Center won a prize for a skill contest in Japan. Some of the graduates are absorbed by the Production Unit of the Center. The program is run by 14 technical instructors and 6 supervisors who have diplomas in engineering. Swedish experts are also working in the project which is expected to be completed in 1985 (Islam, 1978).

Nongovernment programs for the blind

Bangladesh National Society for the Blind (BNSB): The BNSB is setting up a demonstration center which when completed would consist of an eye camp base and clinic, a library and research cell, and a hostel for the blind. BNSB has also set up a vocational training center for the blind in Mirpur, Dhaka with assistance from the West German organization, Christoffel Blinden Mission. Some 110 male and 47 female adults get training in chalk making, weaving, wood work, book binding, light engineering work, jute work, tailoring, braille processing, poultry farming, knitting, and gardening. There are 14 instructors who were trained either at home by visiting experts or in Hong Kong, Bangkok, or India.

Assistance for Blind Children (ABC): ABC's function has been to distribute braille kits to blind children in schools. ABC has also helped in the treatment of blind children through BNSB centers and the Islamia Eye Hospital at Dhaka. ABC has built hostels for blind children who attend the government scheme of integrated special classes in regular schools. It also arranges games, sports, and cultural activities for the blind.

EDUCATIONAL AND TRAINING FACILITIES FOR DEAF CHILDREN

The child with hearing and/or speech defects is in many ways more disadvantaged than the blind child. In a society where charity is a virtue, the blind person can at least take to begging, but the deaf or deaf-mute person who looks normal to others is often taken to be a fraud. Also because blindness is obvious and seems to be more of an affliction, much more has been done for the blind than for the deaf.

Government Programs for the Deaf

Schools for deaf children: The Department of Social welfare runs 7 schools for deaf children. The schools have the capacity to admit 700 children and provide residential facilities for a total of 180 children. The others attend school from their homes. These schools provide eduction up to primary level and instruction in painting and other suitable vocational crafts. There is one school for the deaf in each of the Divisional headquarters: Dhaka, Chittagong, Rajshahi, and Khulna while the remaining three schools are located in the town of Chandpur, Faridpur, and Sylhet.

Training and rehabilitation of the adult: The four schools for the blind and the deaf situated in the four Divisional headquarters are housed in a complex of buildings within the same premises with separate arrangements for the two groups of disabled children. In the same complex are vocational training centers for the deaf, as for the blind. Together, these centers are called Training and Rehabilitation Centers for the Physically Handicapped.

Employment rehabilitation centers: The vocational training center and sheltered workshop for the blind situated in Tongi has similar programs for the deaf in the same complex. The Employment Rehabilitation Center for the Physically Handicapped, as the project is called, trains about 200 deaf children and adults in various trades. In addition to this, there is a Hearing Center which provides various types of services for hearing impaired individuals—e.g. assessment of hearing, diagnosis of type and degree of hearing loss, making of modules for hearing aids, and the repair of aids. Audiologists and speech therapists from Sweden have trained two Bangladeshi technicians to operate the center (Islam, 1978).

Nongovernmental organizations for the deaf

There are 4 nongovernment schools for deaf children managed by voluntary agencies located at Brahmanbaria, Dhaka, Bogra, and Mymensingh. These schools have hostels for boys but the girls have to attend school as day-scholars.

The Bangladesh National Federation for the Deaf has set up a school at Bijoynagar, Dhaka. There are 140 students in the school of whom 60 are girls. There are 17 teachers on the staff; only one of them has appropriate training (received from India). Vocational training in various trades such as tailoring, knitting, carpentry, painting, etc. is part of the program. Unlike blind children, many of whom go for higher education, deaf children rarely proceed beyond the primary level. Emphasis is therefore mainly on vocational training.

FACILITIES FOR THE ORTHOPEDICALLY DISABLED

There are only three institutions that cater to the needs of crippled children and adults; all of them are situated in Dhaka. One institution is run by the government, while two others are run by voluntary agencies.

Government program for the orthopedically disabled

Rehabilitation Institute and Hospital for the Disabled (RIHD): This facility for the orthopedically disabled was started privately in Dhaka by Professor R. J. Gurst, a visiting orthopedic surgeon in June 1972, to treat the freedom fighters injured during the Liberation War. This Institute has been taken over by the government since

1973. Services rendered at RIHD are: orthopedic treatment, including surgery; physiotherapy and occupational therapy; and the production of artificial limbs (braces, walkers, crutches, wheel chairs, etc.). Training programs are available at the Masters and Diploma levels in orthopedic surgery, at the B.Sc. and Diploma levels in physiotherapy and occupational therapy, and at the Diploma level in artificial limb making.

Nongovernment programs for the orthopedically disabled

The Bangladesh Council for Child Welfare runs the Crippled Children's Center. It has a 50-bed hospital, the Feroza Bari Crippled Children's Hospital, named after its founder. There are four trained physiotherapists one of whom was trained in India. The outdoor center provides physiotherapeutic treatment to crippled children. In 1983 alone, 4500 children attended the outdoor center to receive physiotherapy treatment.

A second facility, the Residential Crippled Children's Center, is run by the Women's Voluntary Association (WVA). This center provides residential facilities to poor rural children from outside Dhaka who are undergoing treatment at RIHD. Between 20 to 25 children can be accommodated at a time as boarders. Food, lodging, treatment, and all necessary physical aids are provided free of charge. The center has plenty of rooms and is well staffed with four full time attendants. A supervisor who comes in daily helps with a little formal education of the children. One physiotherapist visits the center daily.

EDUCATIONAL AND TRAINING FACILITIES FOR THE MENTALLY RETARDED

There are not government programs for the mentally retarded who have remained the most neglected and uncared for group in this country until recently. There are two voluntary organizations which run training programs for retarded children and adults. The Society for the Care and Education of Mentally Retarded Children (SCEMRC) which is basically a parents' organization runs 6 special education classes for retarded children integrated into regular schools. Seventy children ranging in age from 5 to 15 years with IQs ranging fron 40 to 70 are enrolled in these classes. These children are trained in the major areas of development—motor, social, cognitive, and communication skills—as well as in some academic skills like reading, writing, and arithment. They are trained also in prevocational skills.

The Bangladesh Institute for the Mentally Retarded (BIMR) was set up as a joint project of SCEMRC and the Norwegian Association for the Mentally Retarded in 1982. Mentally retarded children above 16 years of age are admitted into the vocational training course. After two or more years of training, the students can be transferred to the sheltered workshop. Vocational training is provided in the following areas: home craft, gardening, poultry raising, carpentry, handicraft, and weaving.

Some general education, depending upon the ability of each student, is also provided. A total of 40 students are enrolled in this vocational training class. Tuition fee is charged according to the income of parents. Some of the students enjoy free tuition because they come from poor homes. A small group of severely mentally retarded children with IQs ranging from 20 to 35 are also admitted and given training in basic skills. Thirteen children are enrolled in this group. Twenty-two full time teachers of whom 7 are parents of retarded children work in BIMR and the special classes. The teacher-student ratio is 1:5. In addition, there is a helper in each class. There are two part-time music teachers and one part-time physiotherapists in BIMR. A consultant from Norway supervises the activities of BIMR.

SCEMRC has two more special education schools in Rajshahi and Chittagong and two rural schools in Dhamrai, Dhaka, and Lalmonirhat, Rangpur. About 15 children are enrolled in each of these schools.

In May 1984, a foundation for the developmentally disabled, the Bangladesh Protibondhi Foundation, started its first project, "Kalyani", a school for the mentally retarded (*Kalyani* means blessings, happiness, and progress). Children are admitted in *Kalyani* through the Shishu Bikash Clinic (Child Development Clinic) where they are diagnosed by a psychologist and a pediatrician. So far, 30 children ranging in age from 8 months to 20 years have been admitted. The training includes an infant stimulation program, a program for the severely and mildly handicapped, and pre-vocational and vocational training in cooking, sewing, handicraft, and weaving for the retarded adult. Music, swimming, and gymnastics are also part of the training program.

Counseling of mothers of children who are enrolled as well as those who come from outside Dhaka is a major task of the special education teachers. There are 9 full time special education teachers and one craft teacher. One part-time music teacher and a teacher of gymnastics attend two times a week. A full time principal, trained in special education from the U.S., is responsible for the overall supervision of the activities of the school.

DIFFICULTIES IN PROVIDING SPECIAL EDUCATION TO THE DISABLED IN BANGLADESH

In Bangladesh nearly 50% of school age children do not have access to any educational facilities. The literacy rate in the country stands at 19.7%. There are innumerable priorities for the government to tackle with meager resources. Consequently, the little progress that has been made in the care and education of the disabled is primarily due to the joint efforts of the government and nongovernmental organizations. The following are some of the obstacles that the country is faced with in the development of programs for the disabled:

- lack of awareness regarding problems of disability, not only among the general population but also among educated people;
- lack of concern and interest for initiating programs for the disabled among professionals and policy makers;
- absence of any facility for training of special education teachers and other personnel required to provide effective care and education for the disabled.

From the earlier discussion of the various facilities which exist for the education of the disabled, it is clear that special education teachers and other specialists who are at present employed have either been trained abroad or received brief training locally through resource persons. No organized training program is run by any institution for such a purpose. There are only a few special education teachers and a few physiotherapists who have been trained in India, the United Kingdom, or the United States. There are literally no trained speech and occupational therapists or audiologists in the country. Hence to work for the disabled, one has to pool resources from as many areas as possible. Finally, it can be said that although no easy solution can be suggested at this point, ways and means should be found to more effectively serve the needs of the disabled in this country.

References

Begum, N. (1983). *Case studies of children attending the Child Guidance Clinic of Dhaka Medical College Hospital from 1979 to 1982.* Unpublished Master's Thesis, Dhaka University.

Belmont, L. (1984). *The international study of severe childhood disability.* Interim report prepared for the Bishop Bekkers Foundation Workshops.

Islam, N. (1978). Training and rehabilitation of the physically handicapped. In Dept. of Soc. Welfare (Ed.), *Social welfare services in Bangladesh* (pp. 55-66). Dhaka: Department of Social Welfare, Government of Bangladesh.

Islam, S. (1984). *Children in Bangladesh.* Department of Rural and Community Pediatrics, Bangladesh Institute of Child Health.

Mia, A., Islam, H., & Ali, S. (1979). *Situation of physically handicapped children in Bangladesh.* Institute of Social Welfare and Research, Dhaka University.

Sobhan, M. A. & Rahman, M. (1963). *The disabled child in Dacca.* East Pakistan Council for Child Welfare.

Zaman, S. (1982). *International epidemiological studies of childhood disability—Report from Bangladesh.* Paper presented at the 8th World Congress of the International League of Societies for Persons with Mental Handicap, Nairobi, Kenya.

13

THE DEVELOPMENT AND STATUS OF SPECIAL EDUCATION IN GHANA

S. Walker, K. Marfo, S. A. Danquah, and B. J. Aidoo

Since the 1950s, particularly during the years immediately following declaration of independence from colonial rule (1957), there has been a major thrust to expand educational services. The 1951 Accelerated Development Plan for Education and subsequent legislation—e.g. the Education Act of 1961—reflected the country's perception of education as a crucial tool for national development. Efforts to expand educational opportunities have applied not only to the nondisabled but to the disabled as well (Walker, 1978). In fact, the 1961 Education Act made schooling compulsory for *every child* who attained the school-going age. Thus although no specific special education legislation has been promulgated, disabled children are entitled to education under the 1961 Education Act. Today, largely as a result of strong foundations laid during the early post-independence period, Ghana's rehabilitation and special education services are among the most well developed not only in Africa but in the developing world at large. This chapter traces the development of educational services for disabled children in this West African country and outlines some of the burgeoning problems which need to be tackled if the country's disabled children are to be served adequately and effectively.

Formal recognition of the need to develop services for the disabled dates back to the early 1960s. The 1960 population census and the John Wilson Committee Report of 1960 both pointed to the need for a national rehabilitation scheme. The census showed that there were 148,323 permanently handicapped adults and 10,000 handicapped children below age 15 in Ghana (Amoako, 1975). Sir John Wilson, a blind scholar and Director of the Royal Commonwealth Society for the Blind, had been invited to Ghana in 1959 to examine the needs of disabled persons and to make recommendations to the government. The major recommendations of the Wilson Committee included the following:

- that a national system of publicity and registration be carried out

to determine the size of the problem;
- that special provision be made in schools for the blind and the deaf, but as far as possible crippled children should be absorbed into the general education structure;
- that, as far as possible, the disabled be sufficiently rehabilitated to enable them to be absorbed into the country's normal occupations, both in rural and urban areas, and that specialized segregated institutions should be encouraged **only** where no alternatives existed; and
- that 8 rural rehabilitation units be established across the country (Korsah, 1983).

When Sir John Wilson submitted his report, the government initiated a scheme to provide rehabilitation to as many disabled persons as possible through medical, educational, vocational, and social programs. Today there is a vocational rehabilitation center in each of the regions.

In the middle of 1961 the Department of Social Welfare was formally charged with the responsibility for all aspects of rehabilitation with the exception of medical care. In 1962, however, the Ministry of Education took over the educational aspects of rehabilitation programs and, in furtherance of its commitment to the development of effective services, invited to Ghana two special education experts, R. Howlett and P. Henderson, who were released to the government of Ghana under the United Kingdom-Ghana Mutual Technical Cooperation Scheme. The two specialists undertook a study into the problems of educating handicapped children in Ghana and submitted a report to the government. The report covered general administrative procedures, teacher, primary, secondary, and vocational education, and other matters related to the education of handicapped children (Aidoo, 1982).

The 1960s saw major expansions in special education services and facilities for specific categories of disabled children, especially for the deaf. The increasing commitment that this expansion signified culminated in the establishment in 1969 of a national Headquarters for Special Education within the Ministry of Education. Statistics released by the Ministry of Education (1972) indicate large increases in enrollment between 1972 and 1976. In 1972, for example, a total of 669 handicapped children (blind, deaf, orthopedically handicapped, and mentally retarded) were receiving educational services in 8 schools for the deaf, 2 schools for the blind, 2 hospital schools for children with health and orthopedic problems, and one school for the mentally retarded (Table 1). As Table 2 shows, by the 1975/76 school year this number had almost doubled to 1,144 students, and the number of schools for the mentally retarded had increased to 2, while 2 secondary schools were admitting blind students (Walker, 1978).

The foregoing discussion traces only the history of government involvement in the provision of services for disabled persons; it is important to stress, however, that the history of special education in Ghana goes as far back as the 1940s. In the same way that the introduction of general school education was spearheaded by missionaries long before the beginning of public school education in the 1840s, special education owed its birth and early development to missionaries and to voluntary and philanthropic organizations. In the following sections the historical development of services for three major categories of disabled children receiving education and care is examined.

Table 1. Number of Handicapped Children Receiving Educational Services, 1970/71

School	Girls	Boys	Total
Okomfo Anokye Hospital Sch., Kumasi (health problems)	16	21	37
St. Joseph's Hospital Sch., Koforidua (orthopedic)	4	11	15
Sch. for the Deaf, Wa	8	22	30
Middle Sch. for the Deaf, Mampong	26	56	82
Primary Sch. for the Deaf, Mampong	24	38	62
Demonstration Sch. for the Deaf, Mampong	36	45	81
Volta Sch. for the Deaf, Hohoe	9	12	21
State Sch. for the Deaf, Accra	26	41	67
Sch. for the Deaf, Bechem	34	30	64
Sch. for the Deaf, Cape Coast	6	11	17
Sch. for the Blind, Akropong	30	65	95
Sch. for the Blind, Wa	31	51	82
Sch. for the Mentally Retarded, Accra	8	8	16
Total	258	411	669

Source: Ghana Ministry of Education (1972)

Table 2. Number of Handicapped Children Receiving Educational Services, 1975/76

School	Girls	Boys	Total
St. Joseph's Hospital Sch., Koforidua (orthopedic)	8	3	11
Sch. for the Deaf, Wa	13	33	46
Sch. for the Deaf, Mampong	34	66	100
Demonstration Sch. for the Deaf, Mampong	63	72	135
Volta Sch. for the Deaf, Hohoe	32	48	80
State Sch. for the Deaf, Accra	40	78	118
Sch. for the Deaf, Bechem	59	75	134
Sch. for the Deaf, Cape Coast	31	50	81
Sch. for the Deaf, Sekondi	19	33	52
Sch. for the Blind, Akropong	50	83	133
Sch. for the Blind, Wa	28	60	88
Sch. for the Mentally, Accra	37	69	116
New Horizon Sch. for Mentally Retarded	6	4	10
St. Martin Sec. Sch. Nsawam	2	18	20
Orthopedic Training Center, Nsawam	8	22	30
Total	430	714	1,144

Source: Walker (1978).

EDUCATION OF BLIND CHILDREN

In 1946, the first special education facility was opened at Akropong-Akwapim, mainly through the initiative of Presbyterian missionaries, to provide elementary education in braille for blind children below age 15. Interest in the care and education of blind persons grew during the first few years immediately following the establishment of the school. In 1951 this interest culminated in the formation of the Ghana Society for the Blind as a branch of the Royal Commonwealth Society for the Blind. The goals of the society included the following:

- to awaken interest in the welfare of the blind;
- to spread information concerning methods of preventing blindness;
- to raise funds for the training and care of the blind; and
- to establish or promote the establishment of educational institutions (see Korsah, 1983).

Korsah (1983) reports that "by March 1952, 27 branches of the society had been formed in the main towns" (p. 25) across the country.

Although most of the local branches of the Ghana Society for the Blind did not thrive for long, the society stayed active in the major cities, and in 1954 the society established a vocational center in Accra to train adult blind persons in weaving and basket making. The society also ran two sheltered workshops, one at Bolgatanga in the Upper Region and the other at Nsawam in the Eastern Region.

A second school for blind children was set up in 1958 at Wa in the Upper Region by the Methodist Church. Beginning with an enrollment of 7, the school had a student population of 88 during the 1975/76 academic year. Unlike educational facilities for the deaf which are located evenly across the country, the two schools at Akropong-Akwapim and Wa have remained the only facilities providing elementary school education to blind children. Between 1972 and 1976, however, the combined enrollment of the two schools rose by 25% from 177 to 221 students.

Secondary and post-secondary education: At the Akropong school some secondary and commercial education is available to qualified students. In addition, however, three regular secondary schools, Wenchi, Navrongo, and more recently Okuapeman, have set up programs for blind students. The academic program for blind students is the same as that for regular students and both categories of students take the same final examinations—the West African School Certificate or General Certificate (Ordinary Level) examinations. In fact, Navrongo Secondary School has already produced blind graduates at the Higher School Certificate/Advanced Level General Certificate of Education level, three of whom have gone on to receive Bachelor of Arts degrees at the University of Cape Coast. A fourth blind student recently received a Diploma in the Advanced Study of Education (DASE) from the University of Cape Coast.

Agricultural rehabilitation programs: In 1976 the Presbyterian Church of Ghana and the Christoffel Blindenmission of West Germany set up the Garu Agricultural Rehabilitation Center to improve the living conditions of the blind through some sort of "rural therapy." A second project, the Binaba Agricultural Rehabilitation Center for the Blind, has been set up in the same region under the Anglican Church of Ghana with the support of the Royal Commonwealth Society for the Blind. These two centers provide a suitable rural condition for the orientation of the blind in subsistence cropping, market gardening, and animal husbandry (Dahamani, 1983). Students are given up to three weeks of intensive training, and at Garu there is a follow-up program whereby graduates are monitored for a period of two to three years after graduation to ensure that they are well established.

EDUCATION OF DEAF CHILDREN

Although education of the deaf started some 11 years behind the introduction of education for the blind, it is by far the most advanced area of special education in Ghana, in terms of extent and distribution of facilities. In the year of Ghana's independence from colonial rule (1957), the first school for the deaf was founded in Accra by the Rev. Andrew Foster, an American missionary from the Detroit-based Christian Mission for Deaf Africans (Aidoo, 1982; Aryee, 1973). The goal of the school was to cater for the educational and spiritual needs of deaf and deaf-mute individuals (Aidoo, 1982). Originally named the Ghana Mission School for the Deaf, it started with only 13 students (Aryee, 1973) but grew so rapidly in the first two years that the authorities were forced to find larger accommodation. In 1959 the school moved to Mampong-Akwapim, some 50 km from its original site, where it continued to operate as a private institution under its first Principal, the Rev. Andrew Foster. In May 1962, the government took complete control of the school and it became a free residential school where parents were responsible only for providing their children with school uniforms (Aryee, 1973).

Period of rapid expansion: Following the Howlett-Henderson report and the official take-over of the nation's first school for the deaf, the government sought to set up facilities for the education of deaf children in every region of the country. Consequently the years 1965 to 1978 saw a rapid expansion of educational services for the deaf; schools were opened in Wa (Upper Region), Savelugu (Northern Region), Jamasi (Ashanti Region), Bechem (Brong Ahafo Region), Sekondi (Western Region), Cape Coast (Central Region), Accra (Greater Accra Region), Mampong-Akwapim—Demonstration School (Eastern Region), and Hohoe (Volta Region). Thus by 1978 each of the nine regions of the country had a school for the deaf.

Between 1972 and 1976 enrollment of deaf children in all special schools rose by 56% from 479 to 746. Most of the schools are residential. Through the adoption of a foster parent system, however, the Cape Coast School for the Deaf has maintained a nonresidential approach to education for many years. Under this system about two-thirds of the school's population coming from outside the local community are placed in foster homes. Foster parents receive allowances from the government in addition to subsidies paid to cover the students' evening and weekend meals. Free transportation to and from the school is provided. Brill (1984) cites a presentation by I. K. Nkum in which the latter notes that although there are several problems with the foster parent system, the advantages, in terms of markedly reduced operating costs, far outweigh the problems inherent in foster parenting.

Unit schools for the deaf: The mid-seventies saw the promotion of unit schools for the deaf in Ghana's educational system. Consistent with the policy of integration and normalization adopted by the Special Education Directorate of the Ghana Education Service, unit schools were set up as schools for the deaf attached to a regular elementary school for the purpose of integrating deaf and hearing children. The emphasis for the deaf children in these integrated settings was upon "speech and lipreading as a means of communication" (Odameh, 1977). In September 1975 a unit school was started at Koforidua with two partially hearing and two profoundly deaf children between ages 6 and 8 years. This number had risen to 14 within two years of the unit's operation (Odameh, 1977). During the same period two unit schools were started at Kibi and Adamorabe, also in the Eastern Region.

Early identification and preschool programs: The role of early language and communication training in the development of the hearing impaired child cannot be overemphasized. Successful early intervention, however, hinges on early identification and diagnosis. In Ghana there is a strong recognition by educators of deaf children of the critical role that parents can play in the deaf child's acquisition of language and communication skills during the formative years of development. In 1975 the Special Education Unit started a peripatetic service to run a preschool program and to assist parents to play a more direct and meaningful role in preparing the deaf child for formal education. Dery (1981) has written about the beginning of this program and its emphasis:

> *In that year* (1975), *some experienced teachers of the deaf were appointed to the Regions for the sole purpose of identifying young deaf children, guiding their parents on how to develop skills in language and social training, and eventually*

> *enrolling the children at the school for the deaf in the area. The program has expanded greatly since its inception and continues to do so with the appointment of new teachers each year. It is based on a system of home-visits and the mode of communication emphasized is the use of speech.*
> *... In addition to the work of the peripatetic teachers, schools for the deaf also carry out counseling services in their premises. The emphasis ... is on parents continuing to create and direct learning opportunities at home rather than regarding the program as fortnightly therapy sessions with the specialists. They are further asked to expose the child to a talking environment at all times with a minimum of gestures. Deafness, it is explained to them, only makes learning to speak much more difficult; it does not preclude it* (p. 72).

The program urges parents to provide opportunities for their deaf child to interact with hearing peers. In urban areas, parents are advised to enroll their child at a day nursery for hearing children to promote socialization and oral communication. The program also seeks to educate parents about the use of hearing aids. As Dery (1981) points out, the provision of hearing aids is not a widespread service to children in the preschool program. Parents who can afford hearing aids are encouraged to buy them. However, servicing of these aids is usually done at no charge at the Deaf Education Specialist College at Mampong-Akwapim where there is a qualified maintenance technician.

Dery (1981; p. 73) points out two major problems confronting the peripatetic service program: (a) "the serious lack of amplifying equipment such as audiometers for hearing assessment and speech training units for effective speech development;" and (b) the lack of transportation facilities for a service that involves extensive travelling, a situation which seriously impedes the speed with which peripatetic staff can execute their duties.

Notwithstanding these problems, the program has been largely successful not only in terms of adequately preparing young deaf children for formal schooling but also in terms of promoting parental participation and interest in the education of deaf children. The program has led also to increased admission rates in areas of the country where enrollment has hitherto been low. Unfortunately, however, it appears that existing schools for the deaf are unable to accommodate all children identified through the preschool program. Dery (1981) reports of longer waiting lists for admission; it is hoped that the coming years will see the necessary expansion that will make it possible to enroll all children identified.

Secondary education: For many years deaf students who wanted to receive education beyond elementary school had to leave the country to attend special colleges overseas—e.g. Gallaudet College in Washington, D.C. (Aidoo, 1982). In September 1975 the Secondary/Vocational School for the Deaf was established at Mampong-Akwapim to cater for the needs of academically promising deaf children. Deaf pupils entering this secondary school are exempted from taking the highly competitive national Common Entrance Examination; instead, selection is done through the school's own internal arrangements.

EDUCATION OF THE MENTALLY RETARDED

Current educational services in the area of mental retardation are available mainly to children and youth who are relatively severely or profoundly retarded. Prior to 1970, severely and profoundly retarded children were cared for under a medical model which saw mental retardation as an "illness" or "disease". The emphasis was on medical treatment to the neglect of total developmental needs. The children were usually admitted to the Children's Ward of the Accra Psychiatric Hospital with the frequent observation that they were so retarded that only custodial or skilled nursing care was required. The administration of care, the physical environment, and programming (usually identified as "treatment") were developed along hospital rather than home/school or total rehabilitation lines.

The development of special services and facilities for the mentally retarded began rather late compared to services for the blind and the deaf. While the history of programs for the latter groups was closely connected with missionary activity, the initiative for formal programs for the mentally retarded came from parents of mentally retarded children and from a local voluntary organization—The Society of Friends of the Mentally Retarded. In 1968, the Society started a nursery school for 22 mentally retarded children at the Accra Community Center. In 1970, the Society opened the School and Home for the Mentally Retarded at Dzorwulu, Accra where both day and residential facilities were provided. During the 1973/74 school year the school was taken over by the Ministry of Education with the Ministry of Health taking charge of the health needs of the school.

A second school, the privately owned New Horizon School, was opened in 1972 by Mrs Salomey François, the mother of a mentally retarded girl. The school was first housed in a temporary building, an old church building which was provided by the Roman Catholic Church. In the 1974/75 academic year the school moved into its permanent premises erected through voluntary contributions.

By the 1975/76 school year the total enrollment at the government-supported School and Home for the Mentally Retarded stood at 106 while the privately-run New Horizon School had 10 children (Walker, 1978). Currently 28 children are enrolled at the New Horizon School. A gradual expansion of educational services for the mentally retarded has been taking place over the past few years. In 1977 the Ashanti Regional Branch of the Society of Friends of the Mentally Retarded opened a day school in Kumasi (Marfo, 1977) and in 1983 the Central and Western Regional branches started two new schools in Cape Coast and Sekondi.

Assessment of the mentally retarded: Assessment services have been available at the Clinical Psychology/Behavior Therapy Unit within the Department of Psychiatry, Ghana Medical School since the early 1970s. Between 1971 and 1976 the number of mentally retarded children seen for assessment at the Unit rose from 10 to 15-20 per week. Some parents brought their children to the clinic themselves without referral (i.e. self referrals), while others were referred by private physicians, hospitals, and other paramedical staff (Danquah, 1982).

The medical model of assessment which obtained prior to the establishment of the Clinical Psychology/Behavior Therapy Unit in 1971 was replaced with a developmental model employing a multidisciplinary team approach. Both medical and nonmedical personnel were involved in the identification of the child's mental, physical, educational, and social-emotional needs. The assessment team usually comprised school and clinical psychologists, psychiatrists/physicians, nurses, social workers, pediatricians, neurologists, physical and occupational therapists, and speech, vision, and hearing specialists. Decisions were made with regard to the following: placement in an appropriate educational and/or vocational training program; program planning; and determination of client progress.

During assessment children were classified under three categories: educable, trainable, and profoundly retarded (Danquah, Morson, & Ghanney, 1976). The profoundly retarded children with extensive medical and nursing care needs were admitted to the Children's Ward of the Accra Psychiatric Hospital. Educable and trainable mentally retarded children were recommended for admission to either the Home and School for the Mentally Retarded or the New Horizon School.

EDUCATION OF OTHER "SPECIAL NEEDS" CHILDREN

While blind, deaf, and mentally retarded children are educated and cared for in categorical and segregated settings, orthopedically handicapped children are educated mainly in mainstreamed settings. This practice is consistent with the recommendation of the Wilson Committee that as much as possible children with orthopedic handicaps be educated in the regular school environment. At the Orthopedic Training Center in Nsawam, however, educational services are provided for children who after orthopedic surgery and/or the fitting of prosthetic devices receive various forms of rehabilitation services, including physiotherapy. During the 1975/76 school year, 8 girls and 22 boys with orthopedic impairments were enrolled at the Center. During the same period, 11 orthopedically handicapped children were enrolled at the St. Joseph's Hospital School at Koforidua.

At the post-primary level, St. Martin's Secondary School, also at Nsawam, enrolls students with severe orthopedic impairments. During the 1975/76 school year, 2 girls and 18 boys with various physical impairments were attending the school.

Children with multiple handicaps: There is no facility which specializes specifically in the education and care of children with multiple handicaps. However, in 1978 the Demonstration School for the Deaf at Mampong-Akwapim admitted the first deaf-blind child. Since then a Department of Deaf-Blind Education has been set up at the school through financial assistance from the Christoffel Blindenmission of West Germany. Three deaf-blind children are at present enrolled in the department.

SPECIAL EDUCATION TEACHER TRAINING

One of the recommendations made in the Howlett and Henderson report of 1962 was that further expansion of educational services for handicapped children should rest on the availability of qualified teachers. The rapid expansion of special education services and facilities which took place between the late 1960s and the mid-seventies made it necessary, if not imperative, to set up colleges at home to train specialized teachers instead of relying on overseas training (Dery, 1981). In 1965 the Training College for Teachers of the Deaf was opened at Mampong-Akwapim. At the request of the government of Ghana, the Commonwealth Society for the Deaf seconded Ann Hewitt to the college as the first Principal. Ten years later, in 1975, the Training College for Teachers of the Blind was opened at Akropong-Akwapim.

These two colleges have higher entry requirements than regular teacher training colleges for the preparation of elementary school teachers and are at par, in terms of level of training and specialization, with the Advanced Teacher Training College and the Specialist Training College (both located at Winneba) where subject specialists are trained for the country's second cycle educational institutions. Until recently the minimum entry requirements included possession of a Teachers' Certificate "A" with three years post-qualification teaching experience.

Both colleges offer a two-year intensive program which covers anatomy and physiology, child development, educational and instructional psychology, elements of curriculum development and school organization, as well as specific courses directly related to assessment and program development for deaf or blind children. For example, the program for teachers of the deaf emphasizes speech, audiology, and language and communication, while the program for teachers of the blind emphasizes, among others, braille instruction, mobility training, social competence, etc.

In 1973 the Training College for Teachers of the Deaf admitted for the first time graduates from the universities and the subject specialist teacher training colleges. This change in admission policy, as Aidoo (1982) notes, was in preparation toward setting up a secondary school for deaf students.

Since their inception, the two colleges have functioned beyond the fulfillment of domestic manpower needs; in the spirit of regional cooperation in technical and manpower development, several English-speaking African countries utilize these two training facilities in Ghana. The international role of the colleges dates back to 1970 when, at the International Congress on the Education of the Deaf, Ghana's Training College for Teachers of the Deaf was nominated to serve as the regional center for teacher training in Africa (Dery, 1981). Between 1975 and 1981 the College at Mampong has received students from Nigeria and Sierra Leone in West Africa, Kenya and Tanzania in East Africa, and Swaziland in Southern Africa.

Special education at the University of Cape Coast: At the University of Cape Coast, the country's sole teacher education university, a Bachelor of Education program was established in the early 1970s. Efforts to introduce special education at the Faculty of Education probably began in the 1973/74 academic year but mainly because these efforts were mostly spearheaded by visiting expatriate lecturers, the continuity needed to sustain a special education program was lacking. Up to the 1976/77 academic year the only formal course offering elements of special education was Psychology of Exceptionality, a second-year core course in the B.Ed. program. However, through the Child Development Clinic established in 1974, it was possible for interested students to obtain practical/clinical experience working with exceptional children.

During the 1976/77 academic year a special education elective course was set up for students in the B.Ed., Diploma in the Advanced Study of Education (DASE), and Post-Graduate Certificate in Education (PGCE) programs. Also the first graduate student in special education was admitted at the Master's level during this academic year. Special education is now offered not only to education major students but to students from all faculties wishing to take special education as an elective course. Thus, since 1977 a number of teacher educators with some special education training have graduated from the University of Cape Coast.

The University of Cape Coast is committed to developing the special education area as a major component of the Faculty of Education. Two members of staff are currently receiving further training at the doctoral level in North America. Since 1977, the university has shown active interest in the development and improvement of special education and rehabilitation services in the country. In July 1977, the university teamed up with the Ministry of Education, the Department of Social Welfare and Community Development, and the Ministry of Health to organize the First International Training Workshop on the Education and Rehabilitation of the Disabled. The World Rehabilitation Fund of U.S.A. provided financial support and sponsored several resource persons from the United States to work with local university staff in the planning of the workshop. The workshop has since become a biennial series and continues to receive support from the World Rehabilitation Fund and the three ministries. One of the highlights of the first workshop was the announcement by the Vice-Chancellor of the university that preparations were under way to admit the university's first blind students. In October 1978 two blind students were admitted to degree programs, having successfully completed their sixth form education.

The biennial workshop series opened a new chapter in the university's commitment to the promotion of special education and rehabilitation services not only in Ghana but in Africa as a whole. As Marfo, Walker, and Charles (1983) pointed out in their introduction to the proceedings of the third workshop held in 1981, "The permanent partnership that the workshop series has established between the University of Cape Coast and the three ministries most closely associated with services for the disabled in Ghana should serve as a useful interdepartmental and transdisciplinary model for other African countries" (p. 4).

CURRENT PROBLEMS AND FUTURE CHALLENGES

An appraisal of the present system of providing for the educational needs of exceptional children reveals several problems. First, special education services appear to be restricted to children with the few obvious and perhaps easy-to-identify extreme handicapping conditions—the blind, the deaf, the the severely retarded, and children with severe orthopedic impairments. The system excludes a large proportion of school age children who, although not severely handicapped, physically or mentally, may have difficulties learning at school. Such children may include those with learning disabilities or behavior and/or emotional problems. It is known that high drop-out rates at all levels of schooling constitute a major contemporary problem in developing countries. It is conceivable, as Marfo points out in Chapter 1, that children with mild forms of mental, emotional, and behavioral problems constitute a sizeable proportion of the large number of children who drop out of school each year. There is a strong need to expand special educational services to cover all children who need them, regardless of the degree of handicap.

Second, current programs for the three main categories of handicapped children lack the flexibility necessary to serve each child effectively according to his/her specific needs. For example, a wide range of educational or instructional options should be available to serve subgroups of mentally retarded or visually and hearing impaired children. Existing programs cater primarily for children who fall into the extreme categories of deafness and blindness; hard-of-hearing children or children with low vision, even when they are identified and placed in a special school, are bunched up with totally deaf or blind children and are offered essentially the same instructional program. This problem is not being raised for the first time here; at the International Seminar on Deafness, held in Ghana in September 1972 under the joint sponsorship of the Ghana and the Commonwealth Societies for the Deaf, Aryee (1973) discussed the issue with regard to the anomalous use of manual communication systems with partially hearing children in schools for the deaf.

Third, there is the need to place emphasis upon early identification and early childhood intervention programs. For children who are born disabled or acquire disability early in life, a combination of medical and psychoeducational intervention strategies may prevent such disabilities from causing lasting functional limitations. In this sense, early intervention may serve to reduce future investments in institutional services for the disabled.

The early intervention process should have several components which cut across the jurisdictions of a number of ministries. The screening and early detection components may be undertaken through the Ministry of Health's Community and Public Health Nursing programs with assistance from local community resources such as village or town development committees and school teachers. Other components include the training of Child Development Workers (CDWs) to work with parents and other relatives of the young disabled child to design an intervention program that is appropriate for the child's specific needs. This aspect of the intervention process may be accomplished through a joint program under the Department of Social Welfare and the Special Education Directorate of the Ghana Education Service. The peripatetic service program currently in place for identifying deaf infants and young children may provide a useful model for an expanded early intervention program covering all disabling conditions. Several models and strategies for screening, early detection, and early intervention in the context of Ghana and other developing countries have been suggested in a number of recent works (Fryers, 1981 and Chapter 2 in this volume; Kysela & Marfo, 1983, 1984; Marfo, 1983; Marfo & Kysela, 1983).

Fourth, and related to the last point, is the need to collect reliable statistical data on the prevalence of various disabling conditions upon which decisions relating to the planning and development of special education and other rehabilitation programs can be based. Approaches to the gathering of such data may include the use of the national census and surveys by individual researchers or government departments associated with programs for the disabled. Censuses have been used in the past to obtain statistical information on the disabled population; however, the definition of disabled persons has tended to be limited to the blind, the deaf, and the orthopedically impaired. There is the need to expand the definition of disability and to provide adequate training to census enumerators to undertake this task.

Finally, although Ghana has two of the finest special education teacher education facilities in the developing world, a great deal remains to be accomplished if the country is to serve the majority of handicapped children effectively. Ghana now has four levels of teacher training (Marfo, 1983). The first two levels, Certificate 'A' (Post-primary) and Certificate 'A' (Post-secondary), are basically involved in the training of teachers for the elementary and junior secondary schools. The third (Specialist Training Colleges) and fourth (University of Cape Coast) levels train teachers for the secondary schools, technical colleges, and polytechnics. The University of Cape Coast, in addition, trains teacher educators for the country's initial and post-secondary teacher training colleges. Marfo (1983) summarizes the teacher education problem as follows:

> *In relation to the needs of developmentally disabled children, the disturbing feature of this teacher education system is that no special education component exists at Levels 1 and 2, where teachers for the elementary schools are trained. Special education programs appear for the first time at Level 3, where two specialist training colleges produce teachers of the blind and the deaf. The special education program at the University of Cape Coast, the country's third and highest teacher education institution, which will hopefully lead to positive changes in the coming years, is still in its formative years.* (p. 26).

If Ghana is to meet the needs of its disabled children in every part of the country, the elementary teacher training curriculum should be revised to include courses on developmental disabilities and special education techniques.

An important advantage of a teacher training program that exposes all teachers to special education techniques is that many disabled children who under the present system have to leave their own communities to attend a special school can receive education in their community with their nondisabled peers. Thus, the principle of integration and normalization, which the Ministry of Education supports in principle, will be put into practice. Even more importantly, some of the large number of children dropping out of school because of factors associated with mild forms of developmental delay and/or handicap may be spotted and helped if some form of special education services exist at the elementary school level.

With most teachers being exposed to some form of special education training, a small number of specialists trained at a higher level, such as graduates of the Specialist Training Colleges for Teachers of the Blind/Deaf, can be assigned as regional, district, and circuit special education coordinators and support staff. These specialists would visit schools and assist teachers in identifying special needs children and in developing appropriate programs for them. Regarding higher level teacher training, it is perhaps appropriate to reiterate a recommendation made by participants of the First Training Workshop in the Education and Rehabilitation of the Disabled held at the University of Cape Coast in 1977:

> *The workshop resolved that the various Specialist Courses for teachers of the disabled be combined at Mampong-Akwapim and affiliated to the University of Cape Coast. The resolution called for a three-year course with students reading "general" special education for the disabled in the first two years and specializing in deafness, blindness, or mental retardation in the final year* (Marfo, Aidoo, Archer, Somuah, & Micah, 1977; p. 2).

Of course, other areas of special education—categorical as well as non-categorical—may be included in the training program at appropriate points in the development and expansion of services.

The foregoing does not in any way purport to be an exhaustive discussion of solutions to the problems of special education in Ghana. The authors are cognizant of the many formidable political, economic, and socio-cultural problems that confront the nation. Any realistic reforms and innovations must be placed in the context of these broader problems. The proposals made in this chapter are therefore intended as future challenges that planners and administrators of special education in Ghana should face up to.

References

Aidoo, B. J. (1982). The development and the state of special education services for the deaf in developing countries: A case study and critique. In *Proceedings of the International Congress on Education of the Deaf, Hamburg 1980, Vol. II.* Heidelberg: Julius Groos Verlag.

Amoako, J. B. (1975). *Division of Rehabilitation status report.* Accra: Ghana Ministry of Labor, Social Welfare and Community Development.

Aryee, D. T. K. (1973). The education of hearing impaired children in Ghana. In A. Kamm (Ed.), *Proceedings of the seminar on deafness held in Accra, 1972.* London: Commonwealth Secretariat.

Brill, R. G. (1984). *International congresses on education of the deaf: An analytical history, 1878-1980.* Washington, D.C.: Gallaudet College Press.

Dahamani, E. (1983). Agricultural rehabilitation of the blind in Ghana. In K. Marfo, S. Walker, & B. Charles (Eds.), *Education and rehabilitation of the disabled in Africa, Vol. 1: Toward improved services.* Edmonton: University of Alberta Center for International Education and Development.

Danquah, S. A. (1982). The practice of behavior therapy in Africa: The case of Ghana. *Journal of Behavior Therapy and Experimental Psychology, 13*(1), 5-13.

Danquah, S. A., Morson, J., & Ghanney, E. (1976). Mentally retarded children in hospitals, schools, and home. *Journal Psychopathologie Africaine, 11*(2), 199-207.

Dery, S. E. (1981). Childhood deafness and pre-school education in Ghana. *Educafrica, December* (Special Edition).

Fryers, T. (1981). Problems in screening for mental retardation in developing countries. *International Journal of Mental Health, 10,* 64-75.

Ghana Ministry of Education (1972). *Ministry of Education Report, 1968-71.* Accra-Tema: Ghana Publishing Corporation.

Korsah, K. G. (1983). Integration of health services for the rehabilitation of the disabled in Ghana. In K. Marfo, S. Walker, & B. Charles (Eds.) *Op. Cit.*

Kysela, G. M. & Marfo, K. (1983). Methods and results of early intervention: Home based programs and parental involvement. In K. Marfo, S. Walker, & B. Charles (Eds.) [see earlier reference].

Kysela, G. M. & Marfo, K. (1984). Early handicapping conditions: Detection and intervention in developing countries. In J. M. Berg (Ed.), *Perspectives and progress in mental retardation, Vol. 1: Social, psychological, and educational aspects.* Baltimore: University Park Press.

Marfo, K. (1977). Solving the problems of the handicapped student in Ghana. In K. Marfo, B. J. Aidoo, F. Archer, B. Somuah, & B. Micah (Eds.), *Searchlight on special education: A special issue of the Education Searchlight.* Cape Coast: University of Cape Coast Education Students' Society.

Marfo, K. (1983). Community-based approaches to disability prevention and early habilitation in the context of developing countries. *University of Alberta Center for International Education and Development Occasional Paper Series, No. 2.*

Marfo, K., Aidoo, B. J., Archer, F., Somuah, B., & Micah, B. (1977). Education, habilitation, and rehabilitation of the disabled in Ghana: What future? (Editorial). In K. Marfo, B. J. Aidoo, F. Archer, B. Somuah, & B. Micah (Eds.) *Op. Cit.*

Marfo, K. & Kysela, G. M. (1983). Rationale and strategies for early intervention with handicapped children in a developing country. In K. Marfo, S. Walker, & B. Charles (Eds.) *Op. Cit.*

Marfo, K., Walker, S., & Charles, B. (1983). Toward improved services for the disabled: An African challenge for the 80's. In K. Marfo, S. Walker, & B. Charles (Eds.) *Op. Cit.*

Odameh, E. A. (1977). The Unit School for the Deaf at Koforidua: A report by the headmaster of the school. In K. Marfo, B. J. Aidoo, F. Archer, B. Somuah, & B. Micah (Eds.) *Op. Cit.*

Walker, S. (1978). *The disabled in Ghana: Status and change in information and attitudes.* Doctoral dissertation, Teachers College, Columbia University.

14

EDUCATION AND SPECIAL EDUCATION IN VIETNAM

Marg Csapo[1]

The history of education in the Socialist Republic of Vietnam has its roots in the classic French colonial school system. As with other colonial educational attempts, this system had a number of drawbacks. These include the uneven distribution of the restricted number of schools across the country, favoring urban settings, and the lack of attention to local history and culture. This system of education catered to a small percentage of the population. In 1945 only three out of every 100 children between the ages of 8 and 16 were enrolled in school and only two adults in every 100 were literate (Shmeleva, 1976). The rate of illiteracy among women, national minorities, and people in remote areas stood at 100%.

The development of Vietnamese education is closely connected with the building of socialism (Shi Zung, 1983). The political/economic development of this country from colonialism to socialism bypassed the stage of capitalism. After the withdrawal of the French, the cornerstones of an independent national education were laid (Chyu-Zung, 1977) in Socialist North Vietnam.

The American-Vietnamese war interrupted the economic and cultural development of the country. Many urban schools had to be evacuated and moved to rural areas. The Minister of Education, Van Dong, in 1967 set three tasks for youth:

- to educate themselves at the first, second and third levels;
- to work in industry; and
- to take part in the struggle against foreign invasion.

The work of reconstruction began in 1975 after the termination of military activities.

---

[1]Reprinted, with permission, from B. C. Journal of Special Education, 1983, 7(3), 279-289.

ILLITERACY

The struggle against illiteracy and the renewal of the Vietnamese language (quoc ngu) were among the most urgent goals when the guerilla war against French occupation began in Indo China in 1943. After the revolution in 1945 the Democratic Republic of Vietnam launched three wars: against hunger, foreign invasion, and ignorance. Ho Chi Minh set the task: everyone should be able to read and write quoc ngu (Khoi, 1978). An ambitious scheme was conceived for establishing no less than one class in every village. The motto: "Every literate to teach an illiterate" was based on public good will and masked the real lack of sufficient funds. The eradication of illiteracy became a mass movement: husbands would teach wives, brothers sisters, sisters brothers, children parents, grandchildren grandparents, fathers and mothers their children. It was estimated that 80 to 90 percent of the population of 20 million was illiterate in 1945. Literacy was even lower in the mountain regions where minorities had no written language.

In 1955, one year after the restoration of peace and liberation from French occupation, a three year popular education campaign was implemented. By 1958, 13 years after the launching of the mass literacy program, 93.4% of those between age 12 and 50 could read and write (Khoi, 1978). The large scale literacy campaign mounted an attack on illiteracy on every front. As Khoi (1978) described it, there was propaganda and mass mobilization: books, press, radio, leaflets, slogans, songs, and dances to promote; and prizes, certificates and ceremonies to reward literacy. Courses were organized outside working hours in each hamlet, sometimes for each family. The shortage of schools and materials was solved by scheduling classes in schools, *pagodas* and private houses. Students built their classrooms, used banana leaves to write on, and made their own ink from leaves and fruit. Rapid teacher training courses lasting five to six days helped to promote instruction. Those in the army who could read and write taught others in the army and in the villages.

Literacy training for 3.7 million minorities in the North took longer because in 1945 only the Thai had a form of written language. Vietnamese-related languages of Tay, Nung, Meo and Muong needed written forms. By 1959/60 the Meo and Tay were completed using the Latin alphabet. Eighty five percent of the minority population in the North has acquired a script since 1961 (Khoi, 1978). When South and North Vietnam were united in 1975 there were four million illiterates: 1.5 million women (12-45 years of age) and men (12-50 years of age), 2.5 million children (7-11 years of age) who had not attended school, and old people (Khajapeer, 1979). A campaign to wipe out illiteracy in the South was launched with the same zeal as three decades earlier in the North. Young people by the thousands volunteered to teach others in remote mountain areas or small islands. For the 1.5 million minority population in the South, written language had to be created. In spite of all these odds, illiteracy in the South was eradicated by 1978 (Khajapeer, 1979). Minority groups which form 12% of the population of 45 million are being taught both in Vietnamese and in their own language.

EDUCATIONAL ORGANIZATION

In 1950 schooling was organized in Vietnam at three levels: four years of primary, three years of intermediate, and two years of senior education (4-3-2), resulting in a 9 year educational plan. A standard curriculum was also introduced. New texts in Vietnamese and teacher training demanded immediate attention. By 1958 sixty-three different textbooks and teacher manuals saw ink. In an attempt to bring education closer to the life of the country, students were expected to take part in agriculture and industry as part of their educational training.

After the 1954 peace agreement, efforts were intensified to raise the economic and cultural level of the working people. Evening and correspondence courses organized in factories, plants, and secondary and post-secondary institutions served this purpose. The educational reforms of 1956 established a ten year system, similar to those in other socialist countries. The three stages were four years primary, (7-10 years),three years intermediate (11-13 years), and three years secondary education (14-16 years).

GROWTH OF ENROLLMENT

In the academic year of 1955-1956 there were 716,085 students in schools. Their numbers rose to 2,660,278 by 1964-65 (Shmeleva, 1976) which gave a 25 times increase over a period of 9 years. By 1969-70 enrollment stood at 452,300 in addition to 357,000 students enrolled in national minority schools.

Schools have increased at the second and third levels not only in the valleys but in mountain regions as well. In 1968-69 four school districts in every five had second level schools and every district one

Table 1. Growth in Student Enrollment

Academic Year	No. of Schools
1955/56	716,085
1964/65	2,660,278
1969/70	4,623,000
1978/79	5,855,000

Table 2. Distribution of Enrollment in Educational Institutions in 1978/79

School Type	No. of Schools
Nursery	1,000,000
Kindergarten	1,2000,000
Elementary	2,000,000
Secondary	110,000
Vocational	400,000
Post-Secondary	145,000
Adult Ed. Courses	1,000,000
Total	5,855,000

Table 3. Secondary Vocational Education: Number of Institutions and Enrollment

Year	1975	1978	1980
Institutions	260	265	300
Students	95,500	138,000	147,700

or more of third level schools. In 1967-68 there were 188 secondary schools with 150,000 students. Table 2 shows the breakdown of almost 6 million children and adults in the school system during the 1978-79 academic year as reported by Shi Zung (1982). The growth of secondary vocational education since unification is illustrated in Table 3 while Table 4 displays figures for kindergarten (Ministry of Education, 1982).

TEACHER TRAINING

During the literacy campaign everyone who could read or write was counted on to become a teacher. To meet the needs of the complementary adult education program rapid teacher training programs were given to pupils in secondary schools, skilled workers, and managers to assist the professional teachers with this enormous task.

A core of professional teachers was educated in a formal manner. Elementary teacher training was offered in Pedagogical Secondary schools in 1953. In the following year a college for Teacher Training at the secondary level was opened for national minorities.

In addition to the introduction of universal preschool education in 1960, compulsory elementary education begun in some towns and provinces and in the valley regions in 1961. Teachers were trained in Teachers' Colleges and Pedagogical Secondary Schools in every province to meet the demands created by the expansion of schooling. By 1980 the number of teachers in schools had risen to 430,000 and there were a further 12,000 teachers and paraprofessionals in 44,500 kindergartens whom the U.S.S.R. had helped to train.

EDUCATIONAL GOALS OF THE 1976 PLAN

In 1976 a twenty-year plan for education, enacted by the IVth Congress in Hanoi, set the following objectives for education (Shi Zung, 1982):

- to create a well-rounded new socialist Vietnamese individual;
- to realize education for everyone; and
- to train highly qualified specialists with advanced political knowledge and socialist morality.

Improvement was sought in the efforts to shape the qualities of the new person through vocational education and guidance, and education

Table 4. Kindergarten Classrooms and Student Enrollment

	1975	1978	1980
Classrooms	25,500	40,300	50,200
Students	823,000	1,125,000	1,600,000

Table 5. Number of Secondary and Post-Secondary Students

Year	Secondary	Post-Secondary
1960/61	1,900	11,158
1964/65	26,660	22,371
1978/79	110,000	145,000

to reflect the findings of modern science. Post-secondary education was broadened to meet the needs of society and the professional education of teachers. To realize these aims the enlarging of the network vocational schools was necessary and secondary education was made compulsory. The task of secondary schools was to train workers in cooperation with industrial enterprises so that they possessed vocational, polytechnical skills, academic knowledge, and socialist understanding. Work and study were combined. The aim was to strengthen the cooperation between schools, family, and society and to combine education with the work of industrial enterprises and scientific research. Scientific research centers were set up across the country.

Education was made compulsory from 6-15 years (Grade 1-9). The elementary school aimed to impart general knowledge to prepare the child for active participation in the life of the community, to teach work skills and to prepare for secondary education. A new curriculum and new texts were ready for grade one students in 1980-81.

Secondary education from 15-18 years of age (Grade 10-12) was designed to lead to post-secondary education or work.

POST-SECONDARY EDUCATION

The establishment of the first institute of post-secondary education, the Hanoi University, organized in the manner of French universities, dates back to 1918. Initially the majority of students were enrolled in the Departments of Agriculture, Medicine and Pharmacy. Faculties of Administration and Commerce, Teacher Training College, and schools of Social Work, Veterinary Science, Forestry, Law, and Social Sciences were added. After 1954 much was done for post-secondary education. The College of Pharmacy opened in 1954. Polytechnical colleges offered a number of areas of learning, such as: construction, chemical engineering, mining, electrical engineering. The College of Art and the School of Librarians were among the post-secondary institutions established. Forty professors from socialist countries came to Hanoi University to assist with the expansion.

In 1967-68 there were 33 post-secondary educational establishments in the Democratic Republic of Vietnam with 67,000 students. After the declaration of peace the work of reconstruction and the relocation of schools began. The defence industry, medicine and agriculture, microbiology, and meteorology had attained considerable importance during the war. Now the task was to tie scientific research to the needs of a peaceful economy and industrial reconstruction.

Post secondary education was offered in fifty post secondary schools: four universities, polytechnical colleges, and specialized colleges of agriculture and railway construction. Extramural education and adult education played a major role at all levels through a network of correspondence and evening courses. Secondary and post-secondary education grew very rapidly (Shi Zung, 1980). The growth of secondary and post-secondary enrollment is shown in Table 5.

COMPLEMENTARY ADULT EDUCATION

Once the first level of literacy was achieved the first five year plan (1961-1965) gave priority to complementary education for adults (Khoi, 1978). This system, like the general education system, was divided into four cycles: four years of elementary, three years of intermediate, and three years of secondary education. Grade four education was considered the minimum level for all workers. Theory combined with practice characterized the complementary education courses. Classes were held in government offices, factories, construction sites, and at cooperatives and state farms in addition to schools.

Workers could leave their jobs temporarily on full pay to acquire more advanced education at vocational and technical, secondary or post-secondary schools. The army has developed its own teaching institutes.

SPECIAL EDUCATION

Chyu-Zung (1977) called special education the fruit of economic progress and the advancement of the scientific and technical revolution. In Vietnam special education is relatively new and not widely spread, even though the needs of society have grown greatly since the unification of the country.

In socialist North Vietnam, after the withdrawal of the French, one of the first decisions was the establishment of independent national schools to facilitate the education of exceptional children. However, the post-war economy allowed only for a few experimental residential schools for blind, and for deaf children in Hanoi, Haiphong, Thanh Hoa, Thai Binh and Nam Dinh. In some provinces additional classes were supported by the communities. The general aim of these schools was vocational skill building. The blind were taught Braille and the deaf to communicate. Reading, writing, and parts of the general curriculum that the children were able to learn, were also included. Vocational training was related to local employment opportunities. The U.S.S.R. gave assistance with the establishment of special education, and the preparation of special educators, while the German Democratic Republic helped to equip some experimental schools.

During the same period in South Vietnam special education facilities existed in rehabilitation schools, schools for exceptional children, orphanages operated by religious orders, and some private schools and classes.

In 1975 after the unification of North and South Vietnam the devastating effects of the war presented a dismal picture. In Hanoi the blind formed 0.1% of the population and 1.5% were severely handicapped. In other northern districts, mental retardation was 1%, and children with communication disorders 3-5%. In the South 2.1% of the population were handicapped, 30% of them children.

Table 6 illustrates the percentage of exceptional children in 1973-74 (Chyu-Zung, 1977). To prepare the ground for a unified

Table 6. Categories of Handicapped Children, 1973/74

Type of Exceptionality	Percentage
Paralyzed	33.5
Deaf	8.2
Blind	5.8
Lost one eye	1.9
Lost one leg	5.6
Lost a hand	0.7
Articulation disorders	1.4
Emotionally disturbed	29.3
Mentally retarded	12.3
Other defects	1.3
Total	100.0

special education network the Research Institute of Pedagogical Sciences created a Special Education branch, charged with the task of planning for a special education system appropriate for the needs of Vietnam. The first task was to identify and place students with curable and incurable defects in schools. The war torn economy however, did not allow for universal education of all handicapped children. With no trained special educators, equipment or methods, the country had to rely on the experiences of other socialist countries, adapt them to local needs, and gradually widen the special education network.

In April 1978 the German Democratic Republic invited a delegation from the Ministry of Education to help celebrate the 200th anniversary of the school for the deaf. This provided a rich learning experience. A delegation from the U.S.S.R. and Czechoslovakia came to Vietnam to exchange ideas about special education. The Hungarian People's Republic facilitated Vietnamese participation in the Second Intenational Conference in Special Education which focused on early diagnosis and educational intervention in order to prevent irregular development of the mentally retarded.

Help from various social agencies such as trade unions, women and youth organizations were much needed. Three ministries were involved in special education funding: Education, Health and War-handicapped, and Social Welfare.

The Political Council of the Communist Party recognized the need for classes for the blind, visually impaired, deaf, and mentally retarded at its January 11, 1979 meeting (Minh, 1980). The Research Institute of Pedagogical Science conducted an examination in 12 public school classes and found 31 (5.7%) handicapped children: 27 (87%) mentally retarded, two deaf/hearing impaired (6.5%), and two with speech defects (6.5%) (Minh, 1980). However, a special class set up could only accommodate 13 mentally retarded children due to local difficulties.

The education of the deaf was described by Huan (1980) who mentioned Professor Chan Hyu Tyok who, with his co-researchers, has studied deaf children since 1969 and has established several experimental groups. Their findings point to the need for early intervention under the direction of the Ministry of Education.

The Ear-Nose and Throat Institute of the Ministry of Health, the Research Institute of Pedagogical Science, and the Institute of Rehabilitation Branch of the Ministry of Social Welfare diagnosed 100 cases of deafness among children in 1978. From these 37 were admitted to the Hanoi School for the Deaf. These students were divided into three groups (Huan, 1980):

- The non-verbal 6-9 year old (who cannot hear 80dB through the frequency range 250-1000 Hz).
- 6-9 year olds (who can hear 70-80dB in the range 250-4000 Hz) who can distinguish some vowel and some consonants, and
- 10-13 Year olds from both of the above groups (non-verbal and some with a few words).

Each group is taught by different methods aimed at developing or improving the ability to communicate, as well as impart some general knowledge and vocational training.

The younger pupils are educated for eight years and with the exception of speech, language and literature they follow the regular public school curriculum. The older students receive a five year education program stressing mathematics, natural sciences, history as prescribed in the regular curriculum, and vocational training.

Initially, finger spelling is used to help with understanding and learning. Lip-reading presents some problems with the Vietnamese language. The recognition of each phoneme by the shape of the lips is difficult because Vietnamese has six phonetic signs, which cannot be distinguished by lip movement. The advantages of the language however, are that it has many vowels, among them nine long, four short, and three parallel vowels; there is no declension of nouns, and syntax consists of a relatively stable word order in simple sentences.

Huan (1980) summarized his observations on the education of the deaf:

- There is no schooling provided for several school aged deaf children. Children are admitted usually at 10 years of age or older. The number of well trained educators of the deaf is small. There is no Teacher Training Institute for Special Educators.
- Full cooperation of three ministries (Education, Health and Social Affairs) is necessary to support and organize a well rounded program for deaf children. The model grouping provided by the Hanoi School of the Deaf should be adapted for rural and urban schools and different approaches to teaching should be followed to achieve the primary aim of improved communication (verbal, written, and/or finger spelling).

The number of blind children in Vietnam in comparison with other handicaps is not great. In 1978 only 20 students, between 9-15 years of age were enrolled in the Nguyen Ding Tieu School for the Blind. In the following year another 20 children between the ages of 7-9 years were admitted.

At present, due to economic difficulties, identification with diagnosis is only possible at 5-6 years of age. Another problem lies with the brevity of training teachers of handicapped children receive—only a one- to three-month course.

After thirty years of war, Vietnam is unable to provide special education for kindergarten and nursery school aged handicapped children. There are only a few schools for the deaf under the Ministry of Social and Handicapped Affairs. These schools enroll children at age 10 and provide vocational training.

CONCLUSION

Vietnamese efforts to create an independent, national school system provides an example of the integration of education into the movement of national, social, and economic reorganization. High priority was given to the eradication of illiteracy because teaching people to read and write "awakens consciousness and stimulates participation in political action" (Khoi, 1978). In spite of the lack of necessary economic support, illiteracy was largely eliminated through public participation and the creation of an educational system which catered to children, youth and adults. With assistance from the U.S.S.R. and other socialist countries a rapid increase in all levels of education was made possible. Compulsory education from 6-15 years, grade 1 to 9 is available, and plans are made to include compulsory secondary education. Preschool education has expanded considerably.

Lack of funds, and lack of trained special educators slow down the development of educational provisions for exceptional children. As a result of the war, many children are handicapped physically and emotionally. Services for these children are limited. Vietnam needs assistance to train special educators, develop methods of instruction appropriate for local needs, and funds to build and operate schools for classes for many handicapped children. The need is being recognized, but economic factors and lack of facilities for training special educators keep growth in this area to a very slow pace.

References

Chyu-Zung, N. (1982). *Special education in Vietnamese People's Republic* (Translated by G. Kopeczyk & G. A. Szekszardine). Budapest: Tankonyv-Kiado.

Huan, L. (1980). A suket gyermekek hanoi iskolaja mukodesenek szervesenek, tartalmi munkajanak tapasztalataibol. In S. Kovacs (Ed.), *Korai, felismeres, diagnosztizalas a fogyatekosok iskolaskor elotti nevelese a szocialista orszagokban. A II. Nemzetkozi Gyogypedagogiai konferencia eloadasai.* Budapest: Muvelodesi Miniszterium.

Khajapeer, M. (1979). How Vietnam tackled illiteracy. *Indian Journal of Adult Education, 40*(3), 39-42.

Khoi, L. T. (1978). Literacy training and revolution: The Vietnamese experience. In B. Hall & R. Kidd (Eds.), *Adult learning: A design for action.* Oxford: Pergamon Press.

Minh, D. N. (1980). A rendellenes fejlodesu gyermekek helyzete a Vietnami szocialista koztarsasagban. In S. Kovacs (Ed.), *Korai, felismeres, diagnosztizalas a fogyatekosok iskolaskor elotti nevelese a szocialista orszagokban. A II. Nemzetkozi Gyogypedagogiai konferencia eloadasai.* Budapest: Muvelodesi Miniszterium.

Ministry of Education (1982). *Education in Vietnam.* Hanoi.

Shi Zung, N. (1982). *Sistema narodnoiu obrazovania v socialisticheskoi respubliki Vietnam.* Pyatigorsk: Pyatigorskii Gosudarstvennii Pedagogicheskii Institut Inostrannih Yezikov.
Shi Zung, N. (1983). *Ho Shi Minh Ovacpitanki.* Pyatigorsk: Pyatigorskii Gosudarstvennii Pedagogicheskii Institut Inostrannih Yezikov.
Shmeleva, G. (1976). *Ocherki kulturnovo otpoitelstva v demokraticheskoi respublike Vietnam.* Moskva: Izdatelstyo "Nauka.
Van Dong, P. (1970). Cong tac giao duc va nguoi xa hoi chu nghia. Hanoi

15

THE DEVELOPMENT AND PRACTICE OF BEHAVIOR THERAPY IN DEVELOPING COUNTRIES

Samuel A. Danquah

INTRODUCTION

If the development of human resources in developing countries is to be encouraged, psychological and psychiatric programs must receive more attention. Psychological disorders must be recognized in terms of such effects on the social system as unemployability, absenteeism, lack of motivation, delinquency, crime, drug addiction and alcoholism as well as susceptibility to revolution, violence, and social turmoil. Psychiatric and psychological disorders are chronic conditions which reduce the work force and produce social and economic burdens far greater than is suggested by hospital admission on the basis of severe disorders alone. Psychological disorders may also have serious consequences for the mental, physical, and social well-being of other family members, particularly the children.

However, medical programs in developing countries generally have a much lower priority than programs for industrialization. Psychiatric and psychological programs usually have the lowest priority. Since there are rapid social changes with significantly increasing social stress and unrest, there is a need for preventive and curative measures in the area of mental health. However, trained psychiatrists, psychologists and other mental health professionals are noticeably in short supply in many developing countries. As a result, the focus of treatment is upon pharmaceutical intervention without the necessary psychological interventions.

Once a drug program is established, patients who pose no danger to themselves or to others should be released from existing asylums into the care of their families and at the same time be directed to clinics or community agencies for treatments provided by other mental health professionals such as community mental health nurses, clinical psychologists, behavior therapists, etc. Also community-oriented clinics can be run by a few professionals with the aid of a well trained core of mental health personnel. Such facilities can initiate community and outpatient programs for those with less severe disorders. Again, it is always less expensive to treat individuals in the early stages of their psychological disorders than to wait until complications have developed and psychiatric hospitalization is required. Early preventive measures reduce secondary handicaps and disabilities and hence the number of unproductive and unemployed persons. It appears that now it is possible and economically feasible, through the use of behavior therapists, to develop and improve upon the effectiveness of outpatient programs, mental health clinics, and community mental health agencies.

EFFICACY OF BEHAVIOR THERAPY FOR DIFFERENT PSYCHOLOGICAL PROBLEMS

Behavior therapy has been highly effective with phobic reactions, anxiety reactions (Paul, 1969a), "bed wetting" enuresis (Yates, 1970), stuttering, and ticks associated with Gilles de la Tourette's syndrome (Thomas, 1971; Browning & Stover, 1971). For example, from a review of eighty-five reports of the application of systematic desensitization to nearly a thousand different patients, it was concluded that desensitization could be counted on to produce measurable benefits across a range of distressing problems in which anxiety was a primary concern (Paul, 1969b).

Problems that have shown some improvement when treated with behavior therapy procedures include obsessive-compulsive behavior, hysteria, encopresis, psychological impotence (erectile dysfunction), homosexuality, fetishes, frigidity and orgasmic dysfunction in the female, vaginisimus, premature ejaculation, transvestism, exhibitionism, gambling, obesity, anorexia, insomnia and nightmares.

CHILDREN'S BEHAVIOR PROBLEMS

Also quite responsive to reinforcement therapy are behavior problems of children such as temper tantrums, head bumping, thumb sucking, refusal to eat, and excessive scratching. Promising demonstrations and individual studies have been undertaken with respect to such problems in the home as excessive verbal demands, rebellious behavior, aggressive-destructive tendencies, and sibling rivalry. Other problems outside of the home include isolated behavior, elective mutism, hyperactivity, and difficulties in social interaction with peers. Token reinforcement systems have been shown to be effective in modifying classroom behavior problems such as disruption, failure to study, and low academic achievement (O'Leary & Drabman, 1971). Chronic mental patients have learned a wide variety of appropriate social behaviors after the introduction of a token economy (Paul, 1969b). Studies have shown also that careful implementation of behavioral techniques can produce improvement in the verbal and nonverbal behavior of psychotic and schizophrenic children (Yates, 1970). There is general agreement that psychiatry and mental health programs are benefiting and will benefit further from incorporating concepts and techniques derived from the behavioral tradition.

A report of the American Psychiatric Association Task Force on Behavior Therapy has concluded that the use of behavioral principles in the analysis of clinical phenomena has reached a stage of development where it unquestionably has much to offer informed clinicians in the service of modern clinical and social psychiatry (Aronson, 1974).

DEVELOPMENT OF BEHAVIOR THERAPY IN DEVELOPING COUNTRIES

The heterogenous nature of developing countries makes it impossible to talk about "Third World Behavior Therapy". Countries in the third world are at vastly different levels of development and so are they in the practice of behavior therapy or level of psychological services. Similarly, it is impossible to talk about "African Behavior Therapy." The first Pan-African Psychiatric Congress (1967), held in Dakar, indicated that there were no clinical psychologists/behavior therapists in sub-Saharan Africa (excluding South Africa). Clinical psychology using behavior therapy was first introduced to Ghana in 1971 as a unit within the Department of Psychiatry of the University of Ghana Medical School. It can, therefore, be said that the beginning of Clinical Behavior Therapy in Africa, south of the Sahara, can be traced to Ghana. Undergraduate medical and dental students as well as psychology and nursing students received theoretical and practical training at the Unit. In the area of clinical practice, records showed that there was a continuous increase in the number of patients who attended the clinic at the initial stages of the development of the Unit. For example, attendance in 1972 was 588; eight years later, the number increased to 1751, and during the years 1972 to 1980, the total patient load was 10,256. The Unit and its unique services demonstrated the important role of behavior therapy and its practical relevance in the treatment of psychological disorders in children and adults (Danquah, 1982).

The Unit's goal was not only to introduce this modern technique into the mental health field in Ghana, but also to extend the practice of behavior therapy to other African countries. Fortunately, the first attempt towards this goal occurred in the positive direction in 1982, when the author was appointed (from Canada, Memorial University) by the Nigerian Federal Government to go to the University of Calabar Medical School. It was therefore not until 1982-83, that a Behavior Science and Clinical Behavior Therapy Department was first established at the College of Medicine, University of Calabar. This department was established with the aim that it would follow a similar pattern of development to that in Ghana. It should be noted that there were other departments of clinical psychology in some of the Nigerian universities, such as Ibadan, Ife, and Lagos, offering Clinical Psychology as an academic discipline but not as Clinical Behavior Therapy. While these departments at the Nigerian universities were concerned with the traditional roles of psychological testing and measurements, behavior therapy in Ghana was integrated into multidisciplinary teams which shared clinical and therapeutic responsibilities.

While the development of Clinical Behavior Therapy was taking place in the 1970s in Africa, similar developments were occurring at different periods in other third world countries. For example, countries in Latin America, and others such as Lebanon in the Middle East and Thailand in Asia had started to introduce behavior therapy and behavior modification in their health care practices in hospitals and schools in the 1960s and 70s. In Latin America, behavior therapy has been one of the methods of choice for psychologists since 1970 (Ardila, 1982). It began with the visit of Fred S. Keller to Brazil in the 60s, and following the collaboration of Sidney W. Bijou with Mexican psychologists, behavior therapy was extended to many other countries.

Before the decade of the 70s, psychology and psychiatry in Latin America followed closely the "one-to-one psychiatrist-patient model," but this changed drastically with the arrival of behavior analysis and behavior therapy, first in Mexico and Brazil and later in other countries. A number of laboratories for basic research were opened in

Mexico, Brazil, Colombia, Chile, Venezuela and other countries. Psychiatrists were slower to come to terms with behavior therapy. The majority of psychiatrists still follow the psychoanalytic model or use an eclectic set of techniques, but recently behavior therapy has become an alternative for them. In other countries—Colombia, Panama, Peru, Venezuela, Puerto Rico, Bolivia and Chile— behavior modification was well received and has changed many aspects of psychology and psychiatry. Although psychoanalysis was the main influence around 1970, behavior modification has become an important alternative. At present nobody ignores the experimental analysis of behavior and its application to clinical, educational, industrial and social settings.

Sergio Yulis (1936 -1980) was the leading figure in Chile. After obtaining his Ph.D. in the United States, he went to Chile, where he was instrumental in extending behavior therapy to other Latin American countries. However, due to political difficulties, he left Chile and went to McGill University, Canada as Director of the Clinical Psychology program until his death at a very young age.

In Thailand, no doubt the presence of Mikulas as a visiting Professor at Srinakharinwirot University in Bangkok in 1982 seems to have contributed greatly to increased information about and interest in behavior modification and therapy. Through workshops and public talks as well as visits to clinics and institutions (Mikulas, 1982), it was found that urban clinics were run by physicians whose main approach involved drug and electro-convulsive therapy. These clinics employ some counselors, often social workers and graduates of guidance and counseling. A few psychologists are employed but they do little therapy. The psychologists are primarily used for testing. However, it was found that many Thais are actively interested in increasing the role of psychologically based therapies and practitioners in human services. They recognize the value of behavior therapy as a component of the overall treatment approach.

Thailand is a "developing" country with limited financial resources. It cannot afford many of the time consuming, expensive therapies based on one-to-one long term relationships between a client and a highly trained practitioner. It has been suggested that Thais need to emphasize alternative approaches such as behavior modification, in which a wider range of people (e.g. teachers, parents, paraprofessionals) can be readily trained as change agents, utilizing approaches that can be more quickly implemented and evaluated.

PRACTICE OF BEHAVIOR THERAPY WITH CHILDREN AND ADULTS

The author's experience in Africa (Ghana and Nigeria) suggests that there is visible success in the practice of behavior therapy. The clinical services which were provided at the Behavior Therapy Unit in Ghana demonstrated, for example, successful treatment of phobic conditions—monosymptomatic phobia, frog phobia, sneeze phobia, enuresis, and erectile dysfunction (psychological impotence). Some success has been documented in the area of behavior modification in the classroom and through experimental research on language development in developmentally delayed children (Danquah, 1982). These conditions were clearly or visibly diagnosed and treated successfully, and, as such, demonstrated dramatically the value of clinical behavior therapy in the health program.

According to Mikulas (1983), Thailand is officially over 90% Buddhist and religion has had a very pervasive influence on the people and their culture. He found many commonalities between Buddhism and behavior modification and it is easy and very popular to show the Thais how behavior modification could be approached and practised within a Buddhist orientation (Mikulas, 1982). This seemed to make behavior modification/therapy particularly attractive to many people in Thailand. The Thai government is encouraging the relating of Buddhism to fields such as education and psychology. Monks who have had no formal training have been found carrying out counseling work in Thai rural areas. Training these monks as behavior therapists within their own tradition would certainly enhance the quality of their services.

In Latin America the principle of behavior therapy was centered in educational and clinical problems. In the clinical area of behavior therapy, the new approach competed with psychoanalysis and psychiatry for several decades. It has been indicated (Ardila, 1982) that a number of psychologists and psychiatrists began to apply operant conditioning for the modification of behavior in hospital settings because other approaches had failed. The most successful programs were associated with Sanin's work in Colombia (Sanin, 1977, 1978). As a result, token economy programs were established in Mexico, Venezuela, the Dominican Republic, Ecuador, and other Latin American nations. Other social service areas where behavior therapy has been extended include prisons and homes for delinquent persons. The work done by Dominguez-Trejo (1974) has been recognized as the most advanced work. He used operant conditioning procedures to establish behavior repertoires that are useful inside as well as outside prisons. His work helped to change partially the current situation of delinquent persons in some Latin American countries, particularly Mexico. Canton-Dutari (1984, 1981) was the pioneer in applying behavior therapy techniques in sexual behavior problems. His practical work and research in Panama have received international recognition. Many psychologists and psychiatrists in private practice use behavior therapy procedures.

In Lebanon, the history of behavior modification and behavior therapy began in the 1960s. Clinical psychology/behavior therapy came under the administration of school psychology. School Psychology in Lebanon has a more omnibus character. For example, the roles of guidance counselor, clinical psychologist, special educator and psychometrist are combined. Psychologists are involved in assessment and in a variety of interventions (e.g. behavior modification and psychotherapy), including the treatment of a variety of clients in special education centers, hospitals, and schools. Their work, as indicated in reports (Saigh, in press), was a major contribution to mental health aspects of health care in the nation.

The practice of behavior therapy in Lebanon appears to be similar to the other third world countries. According to Saigh (in press) psychologists in that country render a number of important services. Their work is devoted to the assessment and treatment of a variety of clients in hospitals and schools. Apart from clinical practice, psychology is included in the official curriculum of high schools and universities. This seems to have helped to bring about a more favorable public attitude toward the practice of psychology in Lebanon.

It should be noted that not all third world countries are handicapped by a subsistence economy, or by a total lack of facilities and trained personnel. Some countries do in fact have a developing industrial base and modern medical health systems, and are in a position to implement behavior therapy strategies in psychiatric and mental health programs. What is in great need however, is a coordinated approach to the planning and operation of the program so as to make better use of available talents for practice and for the training of personnel in behavior therapy.

PROGRESS AND PROBLEMS

Behavior therapy and behavior modification grew with the need for a more scientific psychology and psychiatry, and with the opening of new professional centers in several countries. Indications of such growth in the third world included the founding of laboratories of behavior analysis, the establishment of research programs, and the creation of behavior therapy units in hospitals, and in university centers and clinics. Behavioral principles and their application have been used successfully in practically all the reviewed countries in clinical, educational, and social settings.

In the developing countries, behavior therapy and behavior modification have opened up new possibilities for treating clients and patients both inside and outside the hospital setting. Furthermore, behavior therapy in mental health clinics and outpatient settings tends to lend itself more to community oriented treatment clinics designed to avoid hospitalization. Large hospitals are made for more patients, require more psychiatrists and personnel, and are operated at massive costs, tending to perpetuate the same chronic patterns as are already in motion in third world countries. The increasing referral rate over several years to one such clinic program in Ghana (Danquah, 1982) is evidence of positive feedback to an active behavior treatment oriented program. Although the model has been presented in the review with Ghana in mind, the similarities in health systems and infrastructure across Africa, Latin America and other developing countries make it highly applicable.

Since the 1970s, consistent progress has been noted in Latin American countries. Associations for the Advancement of Behavior Therapy and Behavior Modification have been formed. Apart from progress made in the areas of training and practice, Latin American nations have published journals and held series of congresses and conferences aimed at spreading behavior therapy, its research, principles and practices.

The progress of behavior therapy noted in the developing countries is, of course, not without its problems. In Ghana, despite its early achievements in the area of teaching, research, practice and journal publications, the progress has not followed a steady accelerated growth pattern as in Latin American countries. The past few years have been a period of profound political and economic crisis in Ghana. In addition to financial problems, there has been a great deal of criticism directed at health and education systems.

Universities have become centers of conflict and political propaganda. These problems have forced a considerable number of academicians, professionals and others to leave the country. The anti-institutional movement which occurred during this period has affected the universities and the growth of health programs negatively.

The most pressing problems include staffing and training. There is a need for qualified personnel to practice and to teach; but this requires commitment on the part of government to devote more resources to mental health. Behavior therapy, if supported, could play a major role in reducing the high cost of caring for patients in poorly staffed custodial institutions. The promotion of behavior therapy could also enhance the provision of effective mental health services to schools, clinics, hospitals, and other social service areas. In the area of research, the Ghanaian model can serve as a natural laboratory for other African countries and as a base for cross-cultural research, especially its emphasis on multifaceted research into etiology and traditional beliefs and healing practices.

Behavior therapy and behavior modification have proved successful by teaching parents, teachers, nurses and other health personnel to assist people in coping with the characteristic stresses of the culture. Through behavioral techniques, the above mentioned personnel in the developing countries are well equipped to deal with a variety of behavior disorders that have become the domain of psychiatry but which, in fact, are not mental illnesses.

Behavior therapists in Ghana have also worked successfully with traditional healers who assist in reintegrating the patient into the community. Successful treatment can be explained in terms of traditional and cultural beliefs along with the concurrent use of indigenous therapies. Where these are not counterproductive, it is good sense not to oppose them. Indeed, certain existing traditional healing practices may be useful. Channelling clients' floating anxieties into phobic reactions becomes more manageable with behavior therapy techniques. Behavior science functions to explain *how* a given condition occurs, while witchcraft explains *why* the process occurs, or why it occurs in one individual and not in another. A behavior therapist working in such a specific cultural environment needs to rely on cross-cultural research to gain more familiarity with cultural practices that may have relevance for the behavior therapy approach. At the moment this is a problem facing behavior therapy in developing countries. Very little has been done in this direction; therefore there is need for a body of research on the effective application of behavior therapy in cross-cultural contexts. Only through such research can the benefits of this approach be maximized for the majority of the people in the developing countries.

Another problem which needs mention here is the negative attitude of some of the psychiatrists in Africa—mainly those who are pharmaceutically oriented and have psychodynamic training—toward the practice of psychology and traditional treatments. This kind of opposition constitutes a major hindrance to the smooth development of behavior therapy. The introduction of behavior therapy programs into developing countries requires considerable effort, if the inertia on the part of the government and local administration is to be overcome. Conferences, workshops, symposia, etc. on behavior therapy in the third world are very important at this stage. It is less than 15 years since behavior therapy was first introduced in the third world. Psychiatrists and psychologists working in the field are in the minority. However, with the current increased emphasis on the teaching of behavior therapy to medical, psychology, social work, and nursing students, we should look forward to greater activity in the near future.

SUMMARY

The issues considered in this review of behavior therapy in developing countries are of utmost importance to all experts who are involved in planning to introduce behavior therapy in other developing countries. We have discussed how a given culture's concept of health may significantly influence its acceptance of certain practices. Ill-health may be attributed to supernatural forces, taboos, and violations of customary practices. It seems more advisable, therefore, to deal with traditional healers who reinforce these beliefs without trying to change them. Research in several developing countries—e.g. Ghana, Thailand, and some Latin American countries—has demonstrated how helpful it would be to incorporate traditional healing concepts into some parallel or collaborate systems of treatment. In other words, the expert in behavior therapy should explore ways in which beneficial elements of traditional healing practices may be incorporated into comprehensive modern treatment programs.

Great progress has been made in some of the third world countries, whereas in others like Lebanon and Thailand, there is rather slow but, nevertheless, noteworthy progress. In Africa, apart from Ghana and a few states in Nigeria, behavior therapy has not been integrated into mental health programs.

In general, the topics covered by this review testify to the enthusiasm of third world behavior therapy pioneers and to their eagerness to keep and expand the training of behavior therapists in the third world. Given limited financial resources, educational and training programs for personnel in developing countries, behavior therapy should, in the long run, prove to be a more profitable investment than existing custodial mental health systems.

References

Ardila, R. (1982). International developments in behavior therapy in Latin America. *Journal of Behavior Therapy and Experimental Psychiatry, 13*(1), 15-20.

Aronson, J. (1974). *Behavior therapy in psychiatry: APA Task Force Report (Report 5).* Washington: American Psychological Association.

Browning R. M. & Stover, D. O. (1971). *Behavior modification in child treatment.* Chicago: Aldine-Atherton Publishers.

Canton-Dutari, A. (1981). Ejaculacion prematura: Terapia de control sin parej. *Rev. Latinoam Psico., 13,* 111-114.

Canton-Dutari, A. (1984). The treatment of homosexuality: A model for controlling active homosexual behavior. *Archives of Sexual Behavior, 3,* 367-372.

Danquah, S. A. (1976). A preliminary survey of beliefs about severely retarded children in Ghana. *Journal Psychopathologie Africaine, 12*(2), 189-199.

Danquah, S. A. (1982). The practice of behavior therapy in Africa: The case of Ghana. *Journal of Behavior Therapy and Experimental Psychiatry, 13*(1), 5-13.

Dominguex-Trejo, B. (1974). Contingencies aplicables al control de grupos instucionalizados. In R. Ardila (Ed.), *El analisis experimental del comportumiento, la contribucion Latino-Americana.* Mexico: Editorial Trillas.

Harding, T. Q. (1977). Mental health research in Africa. *African Journal of Psychiatry, 3*(182), 46-56.

Mikulas, W. L. (1982). Buddhism and behavior modification. *Psychological Records, 31,* 331-342.

Mikulas, W. L. (1983). Thailand and behavior modification. *Journal of Behavior Therapy and Experimental Psychiatry, 14*(2), 93-97.

O'Leary, K. D. & Drabman, R. (1971). Token reinforcement programs in the classroom: A review. *Psychological Bulletin, 75*, 379-398.

Paul, G. L. (1969a). Outcome of systematic desensitization: II. Controlled investigation of individual treatment, technique variations, and current status. In C. M. Franks (Ed.), *Behavior therapy* (pp. 105-159). New York: McGraw-Hill.

Paul, G. L. (1969b). Chronic mental patients: Current status, future directions. *Psychological Bulletin, 71*, 81-94.

Saigh, P. A. (In press). School psychology in Lebanon. *Journal of School Psychology.*

Sanin, A. (1977). Salud mental y enfermedad mental. *Rev. Latinoan Psicol., 9*, 337-339.

Sanin, A. (1978). Economia de fichas en un hospital psiquiatrico. *Rev. Psicol Clin. (Peru), Special Issue,* 32-39.

Thomas, E.J. (1971). Self-monitoring and reciprocal inhibition in the modification of multiple tics of Gilles de la Tourette's syndrome. *Journal of Behavior Therapy and Experimental Psychiatry, 2,* 159-171.

Yates, A. J. (1970). *Behavior therapy.* New York: John Wiley & Sons.

PART THREE: SOCIAL-PSYCHOLOGICAL CONSIDERATIONS

16

ATTITUDES TOWARD THE DISABLED AS REFLECTED IN SOCIAL MORES IN AFRICA

Sylvia Walker

DISABILITY: A CROSS CULTURAL VIEW

Man is continuously striving to come to terms with his environment in order to ensure safety and maintain life (DeGraft-Johnson, 1970). Disability and concerns about illness are inevitable in every society. These phenomena, with their socio-cultural, biological, and economic implications, have disruptive effects on social relationships (Amorin, 1971; Walker, 1981). Parsons (1951) points out that the birth and rearing of a child constitute cost to the society through pregnancy, childcare, socialization, formal training and other channels, since time and energy are expended. Disability may be perceived as preventing the individual from playing out his/her full social role, thereby giving only a partial return for this cost. (Is partial return for the cost of "rearing" the only source of social loss when an individual is disabled?)

> *We may say that illness is a state of disturbance in the normal functioning of the total human individual, including both the state of the organism as a biological system and of his personal and social adjustments. It is thus partly biologically and partly socially defined. Participation in the social system is always potentially relevant to the state of illness, to its etiology and to the conditions of successful therapy, as well as other things.* (Parsons, 1951, p. 431)

All societies, both modern and ancient, have developed both programmatic and philosophical ways of coping with the problems of health and disability (Nukunya & Twumasi, 1973). The history of medicine is primarily an account of man's endeavors to conquer disease and the effects of handicapping conditions (Amorin, 1971). As stated by Parsons (1951), illness and disability interfere with social obligations. The nature and degree of the disturbance determine the social group affected, i.e., the immediate family, the extended family, lineage group, clan, or even the entire community. Health and wholeness are cherished. Therefore, society takes what are considered as legitimate actions to normalize conditions. Methods taken to preserve and restore physical well-being throughout the ages have been dictated by prevailing concepts of disease causation (Pappoe, 1973; Twumasi, 1975). Amorin (1971) examined the evolution of perceived causes of illness and disability and discussed strategies used to maintain and regain physiological stability. In addition to natural causes such as the germ theory, man has conceptualized disability and disease as being the result of sin (failure to keep a taboo or religious code), evil influences (e.g. devils, demons, witches) or supernatural forces such as the ancestors.

Concepts of supernatural causation of disease are not unique to Africa. These concepts have persisted in Europe, Asia and America side by side with other concepts and they still exist to varying degrees in both western and nonwestern societies (Amorin, 1971; Walker, 1978). Fiscian (1972) feels that significant differences in theories concerning disease causality between African and Western man are a matter of degree, not kind. He observes also that since man is complex rather than simplistic in thinking, individuals and groups are neither wholly abstract nor concrete, analytical nor emotional. Rather, mankind is conceptually dualistic. Most superstitious beliefs do in fact possess a logical and an internal consistency of their own and are not any less logical than explanations in terms of destiny, fate or the Christian God. As a result of the dual nature of man's thinking, even when natural causes for disability and illness are recognized, human beings, across cultures, combine efforts to maintain biological stability with attempts to appease the supernatural. Pappoe (1973) makes the point that African concepts of health and disease are frequently viewed in isolation. As a result, a disproportionate amount of emphasis is placed on beliefs in the supernatural as if these beliefs were characteristic of Africa alone.

Before discussing research related to attitudes toward the disabled as reflected in societal mores in Africa, it is necessary to explore at least some of the factors which shape these practices. Nukunya, Twumasi, and Addo (1975) suggest that the key to comprehension of African societies is to be found in the importance of kinship, which in many societies is articulated in corporate descent groups, extended families, and extensive kinship networks. Related to these are emphases on group solidarity, respect for age, and reverence for ancestors. The rules which govern these institutions and practices stipulate that their violation will bring disaster to both the culprit and his/her close relatives. The visible signs which indicate that an offense has been committed are the misfortunes which occur.

CULTURAL CLIMATE AND CONCEPTS ABOUT DISABILITY AND MISFORTUNE

All over Africa, and in fact universally, significant ceremonies and rituals are to varying degrees performed at the three major turning points in an individual's life. In traditional societies, these rites are collectively termed *Rite de Passage* (Rites of Passage from one stage to another). The crucial transition points are generally the time when a person enters the world through birth, when he/she comes of age and enters the world of the adult, and when through death he/she departs from this world and enters the world of of the forebears. The latter is of particular importance in many African cultures because of the esteem held for the ancestors. Not everyone is accorded this esteem, however. Rites of Passage signify full membership in the society and full acceptance in a clan structure. They are expressed by observance of ritualistic ceremonies (Forster, 1973; Sarpong, 1974). Sarpong (1974) observes that persons who have not fulfilled their full obligations to the society such as bearing offspring and those who die from suicide are generally not accorded the status of full adulthood. It is likely that among some groups, individuals with obvious handicapping conditions are also excluded from full adult status.

Another vital aspect of the African cultural climate is the importance of religion. Ewusie (1968) states that religion is man's attempt to interpret the universe in spiritual terms. Sarpong (1974) describes this complex belief system through application of Parinder's Triangle Theory:

> *At the apex is God, the supreme and creator spirit. The two sides of the triangle are the lesser deities and ancestors, both important and one made more of than another in varying places. The base of the triangle is composed of those beliefs and practices often called magical* (Sarpong, 1974, p. 44).

While the lesser deities (i.e. earth and river gods or goddesses) and esteem for the ancestors are important aspects of religious beliefs in Africa, the degree of their importance varies from one social group to another.

Belief in witchcraft is prevalent in Africa. It is the concept of some supernatural power by which an individual may become possessed and which is used predominantly for evil purposes (Dodu, 1975; Enyan, 1977; Middleton, 1967; Walker, 1978). Forster (1973) states that persons who say that they are responsible for the death of children and other misfortunes often use confessions to witchcraft as a means of expressing unconscious guilt feelings.

Societies in Africa as elsewhere enforce taboos as a means of regulating individual and group behavior. "The word taboo is derived from a Polynesian term *tabu* which means forbidden and can be applied to any sort of probibition" (Sarpong, 1974, p. 51). Specific taboos vary from one lineage group to another. However, they generally direct members of the group to refrain from immoral behavior and to abstain from certain foods and other practices. Amorin (1971) makes the point that certain taboos in most communities are very old, since they have been accepted and observed for centuries. To a certain extent taboos played a role in determining social relationships. Among some groups it is believed that an ancestral spirit may provoke illness or disability as punishment for not abiding by a taboo. When illness or disability occurs, the family generally searches for the reason for the presence of such a disaster. An individual may break a taboo unintentionally; he/she may not even have been aware of an offense until he is told of it because, as Sarpong (1974) points out, "Culture is learned ... it does not depend on inborn instincts or reflexes, or any other biologically inherited forms. It is almost wholly the result of social invention" (p. 7).

VARIATIONS IN BELIEFS ABOUT DISABILITY IN AFRICA

During the process of growing up, the African child becomes acquainted with the aspects of these mores and beliefs as they apply to his/her own subculture. The individual is socialized through various customs and value systems (Field, 1962; Forster, 1973; Kaye, 1962). A child growing up among the Ngwas of Nigeria for example, would be taught to accept the strong belief in ghosts. The Ngwas are convinced that the spirits of their loved ones and their enemies come from the spirit world in order to inflict punishment. It is maintained that if a person dies and the offspring do not give him/her a befitting burial, he comes back to earth to harm them in one way or the other. Anyatunwa (1977) reports of being told as a child that a neighbor was deaf because he had not given his father an appropriate funeral.

Pappoe (1973) cautions against assuming homogeneity of African customs and attitudes toward disease. Many surveys of African concepts of illness and disability do not give respondents ample opportunity to identify natural processes as the genesis of these conditions (Adams, 1949; Pappoe, 1973). Many Africans do attribute disease to natural origins. Some see a combination of both natural and supernatural etiology (Dodu, 1975; Twumasi, 1975). Perhaps more important than the reasons given to explain ill-health and disability is the fact that much emphasis is placed on the social implications of these conditions (Nukunya et al., 1975).

An examination of research related to attitudes toward the disabled in Africa gives insight into the effects of tradition and custom as well as the status of various disability groups within some specific settings. In a study of beliefs among the Ngwas of the Imo State in Nigeria, Anyatunwa (1977) found that Albinos and the physically handicapped are thought to have sinned in their previous lives. This position is based on a strong belief in reincarnation. It is also held that a person must do everything possible not to evoke the anger or disfavor of parents or old men and women, since the consequence is a curse upon the individual or his/her family.

> *You dare not mock anybody that is disabled so that he might not curse you, because it is believed that the curse will have repercussions on the cursed when he is reincarnated* (Anyatunwa, 1977, p. 5).

In addition to the recognition of the effect of heredity, there is also a strong belief among the Ngwas in evil spirits and the power of sorcery (Nnabagwu, 1977). While deafness and blindness are seen as hereditary conditions, deafness is also viewed as a means whereby a person may work off his/her *Karma.*[2] Women who give birth to children with handicaps are believed to have been charmed by sorcerers. However, the children are regarded as having been wicked in their former lives.

---

[2](Sins). It is possible that some similarity may be found between the utilization of this concept of *Karma* among the Hindus and among the Ngwas of Nigeria.

After examination of attitudes among another Nigerian group, the Yorubas, Adeoke (1977) ascertained that many disabilities are perceived to be the work of wizards as punishment of offenses. In addition to pointing out other explanations for the presence of disability (i.e. the presence of foreign bodies such as lizards, the work of a local deity), Adeoke (1977) also reports unique conceptualizations among the Yoruba people as to which conditions are categorized as disabilities. His findings suport the observation made by Lippman (1972) that deviance is an attribute defined by society rather than an innate characteristic of the individual. Having a goiter is a disgrace, since it is felt by many to be a punishment. On the other hand, hydrocephalus is not regarded as a disability, and thus there is no stigma attached to it. Epilepsy (felt to be caused by the presence of lizardlike creatures in the stomach) is believed to be contagious. Physical handicaps are seen by many as the work of a special deity. The following account is given of the origin of beliefs related to the physically impaired among the Yoruba:

> *Orisannla was believed to be the sculptor divinity. He has been given the prerogative to create man as he chooses. He makes men of shapely or deformed features. Hunchback, albinism and crippling conditions are regarded to be special marks of his prerogative either signifying his displeasure at the breach of some taboo or to show that he could act as he likes* (Adeoke, 1977, p. 6).

Among some Yorubas, blindness is perceived as being caused by black magic as the result of jealousy.

A survey of attitudes towards disease and disability among Rhodesian medical trainees was conducted by Adams (1949). The subjects represented the following ethnic groups: Mambwe, Lygu, Usho, Mwinimwanga, Nsenga, Tumbuka, Besa Tabwa, Chishega, Ila and Lozi. The 43 students in the sample indicated that people in their communities believed, to varying degrees, in both natural and supernatural influences on illness and disability. Seventy percent stated that their lineage group held supernatural influences to be the etiology of disease and disability. Thirty-four percent indicated that traditional doctors could prevent disease and 33% were of the opinion that traditional medical procedures were superior to scientific methods. Analysis across ethnic groups suggested a number of similarities between these concepts and those of other Africans. For example, cerebral palsy was seen as being caused by either witchcraft and spirits or by failure to observe a taboo. Blindness was attributed to witchcraft; leprosy was perceived as being the result of witchcraft, spirits, or natural causes.

Nukunya and his colleagues (1975) cited other variations in the response to the supernatural in Africa as it related to disability and sickness:

> *Such forces are many and vary from society to society. Among the Azande, for instance, witchcraft may be held responsible. In Northern Ghana among the Talensi, it is believed that no one may die without the approval of the ancestors who in some appropriate cases themselves initiate sickness leading to death. Among the Mende of Sierra Leone supernatural forces associated with secret societies may cause madness, barenness, etc. Yet among the Ewe of Ghana and Togo, though the ancestors, cult groups, and witches feature prominently in these considerations, most deaths and sickness are put down to work of sorcerers* (Nukunya et. al., 1975, pp. 116-117).

Although the literature contains a number of references to concepts of supernatural etiology of disability, researchers state that natural causes are also recognized among Africans (Dodu, 1975; Pappoe, 1973; Twumasi, 1972a,b, 1975). In general, it is believed that natural causes are remediated by either scientific or traditional (herbal) medicines.

In addition to modern medical personnel, most African societies contain a number of persons skilled in traditional medicine, psychology and occultism. Specific titles for such individuals vary from one society to another; however, they include traditional healer/doctor (among them herbalists and bonesetters), juju men, diviners and fetish priests and priestesses, all of whom are trained to practice their skills (Brookman-Amissah, 1975; Twumasi, 1972a,b).

When physical and mental misfortunes are perceived as being the consequence of supernatural forces, the supernatural is engaged through employing the services of diviners, etc., as a means of eliminating the condition (Field, 1962; Nukunya et. al., 1973; Walker, 1978). Remedial steps taken are related to perceived causes. Agents who are consulted to alleviate disability and sickness are as varied as the perceived causation.

IMPLICATIONS FOR THE PROVISION OF SERVICES TO THE DISABLED IN AFRICA

The foregoing literature provides an overview of the influences of tradition and custom on attitudes toward the disabled in select settings in Africa. Research conducted by Danquah (1977) and Walker (1978, 1983a) indicated that disability is frequently associated with uncomfortable and distressing circumstances. For example, a control group study conducted in Africa by Walker (1982) revealed that (in spite of the fact that attitudes were generally positive) post-test scores for the control group showed less positive attitudes towards the deaf than were revealed during the pre-test. A possible explanation for this shift in a negative direction by control group subjects could have been that participation of this group in the study may have aroused dissonance within the cognitive and affective attitude components without providing resolution of such tensions.

A study which compared the attitudes of college students and non-students toward the disabled in Ghana (Walker, 1981) revealed significant differences in attitudes of these groups toward the disabled. While overall attitudes were generally positive for both groups, non-students tended to blame the disabled for the presence of a handicapping condition more than did students. Non-students placed greater emphasis on occurences, such as nonobservance of a taboo, as the cause of disability than did students. Findings from this study which included questions focusing on the value of educating and training the mentally retarded, suggested that students were more optimistic about the potential of the mentally retarded than were non-students. However, an examination of findings related to social competence and interaction of the disabled with the non-disabled revealed greater similarities in the responses of students and non-students. In both instances, attitudes were less positive toward the disabled. A sizeable number of respondents in both groups were reluctant to have their offspring associate with the mentally retarded. (Eighteen percent of the students and 16% of the non-students agreed with the statement: "Blind people and normal people can't really understand each other."

In spite of the heavy influence of tradition and culture on the formation of attitudes toward illness and disability in Africa, it cannot be assumed that all or the majority of these attitudes are negative or harmful. Attitude studies conducted by the author in West Africa revealed on one hand considerable variation in attitude toward the handicapped and on the other hand considerable positive and/or supportive approaches concerning the needs of the disabled (Walker, 1981, 1982, 1983a,b).

It must be noted that in recent years a sizeable number of countries in Africa, as in other parts of the globe, have had to face substantial economic, environmental, and political challenge (Marfo, Walker, & Charles, 1983). Therefore, strategies to assist and improve the status of the disabled must be developed within a context which seeks to maximize the potential of both the disabled and non-disabled (Walker, 1983b).

A major implication of the literature and research reported in this review is the need for coordinated effort in research and program development with respect to disabled persons in developing countries. Social agencies and universities in and outside of Africa are presented with a strong challenge regarding the special education and rehabilitation needs of the disabled. It is recommended that the many resources available through international bodies such as UNESCO and leading institutions of higher education in the United States and Europe be marshalled and combined with similar resources available at institutions such as the University of Cape Coast (Ghana) and the University of Ibadan (Nigeria) to respond to the personnel training, societal education, health care, and program development needs in Africa, Asia, and similar areas to facilitate equal opportunity for the disabled.

References

Adams, P. C. G. (1949). Disease concepts among Africans in the Protectorate of Northern Rhodesia. *Rhodes-Livingstone Journal, 10*, 14-50.

Adeoke, E. O. (1977). *Yoruba attitudes toward the disabled.* Unpublished Essay (required for Certificate in Special Education), University of Ibadan, Nigeria.

Amorin, J. K. E. (1971). *Concepts of disease causation throughout the ages.* Accra: Ghana Universities Press.

Anyatunwa, Z. A. (1977). *A study of beliefs among the Ngwas in Imo State.* Unpublished essay (required for Certificate in Special Education), University of Ibadan, Nigeria.

Brookman-Amissah, J. (1975). *The traditional education of the indigenous priesthood in Ghana.* Faculty of Education Occasional Paper, University of Cape Coast, Ghana.

Danquah, S. A. (1977). *A preliminary survey of beliefs about severely and moderately retarded children in Ghana.* Paper presented at the First Training Workshop in the Education and Rehabilitation of the Disabled, University of Cape Coast, Ghana.

DeGraft-Johnson, K. E. (1970). *Proceedings: Ghana Academy of Science.* Accra: University of Ghana Press.

Dodu, S. R. A. (1975). Meeting the health needs of developing countries. *Universitas, 5(1)*, 3-16.

Enyan, K. (1977). Witch turned into monkey. *Palaver-Tribune, April 13-19.*

Ewusie, J. Y. (1968). *Science and religion.* Cape Coast: University of Cape Coast.

Field, M. J. (1962). *Search for security: An ethno-psychiatric study of rural Ghana.* Chicago: Northwestern University Press.

Fiscian, C. E. (1972). Cognition and superstition. *Universitas, 1(4)*, 79-82.

Forster, E. F. B. (1973). *The basic psychology and psychopathology of the African peoples.* Accra: Ghana Universities Press.

Kaye, B. (1962). *Bringing up children in Ghana.* London: George Allen and Unwin Ltd.

Lippman, L. (1972). *Attitudes toward the handicapped.* Springfield, Illinois: Charles C. Thomas.

Marfo, K., Walker, S., & Charles, B. (1983). Toward improved services for the disabled: An African challenge for the 80's. In K. Marfo, S. Walker, & B. Charles (Eds.), *Education and rehabilitation of the disabled in Africa, Vol. 1: Toward improved services.* Edmonton: University of Alberta Center for International Education and Development.

Middleton, J. (1967). *Magic, witchcraft and curing.* Austin, Texas: University of Texas Press.

Nnabagwu, N. O. (1977). *A study of beliefs about disabilities among the Ibos (Ngwas).* Unpublished Essay (required for Certificate in Special Education), University of Ibadan, Nigeria.

Nukunya G. R. & Twumasi, P. A. (1973). *Traditional attitudes towards health, disease and family planning in four selected communities in Ghana.* (PDP Research Project #2) Accra: Institute of Social Science and Economic Research.

Nukunya, G. R., Twumasi, P. A. & Addo, N. O. (1975). Attitudes towards health and disease in Ghanaian society. *Conch, 7(1&2)*, 113-136.

Pappoe, V. L. (1973). *Ghanaian traditional concept of disease and medical practices.* Unpublished doctoral dissertation, Yale University School of Medicine.

Parsons, T. (1951). *The social system.* New York: The Free Press.

Parsons, T. & Bales, R. F. (1955). *Family: socialization and interaction process.* New York: The Free Press.
Sarpong, P. (1974). *Ghana in retrospect: Some aspects of Ghanaian culture.* Accra-Tema: Ghana Publishing Corporation.
Twumasi, P. A. (1972a). Ashanti traditional medicine and its relation to present day psychiatry. *Transition, 41,* 50-62.
Twumasi, P. A. (1972b). Medicine: Traditional and modern. *Insight and Opinion, 7*(1), 20-50.
Twumasi, P. A. (1975). *Medical systems in Ghana; A study in medical sociology.* Accra: Ghana Publishing Corporation.
Walker, S. (1978). *The disabled in Ghana: Status and change in information and attitudes.* Doctoral dissertation, Teachers College, Columbia University.
Walker, S. (1981). Cross-cultural variations in the perception of the disabled. *International Journal of Rehabilitation Research, 4,* 90-92.
Walker, S. (1982). A comparison of the attitudes and knowledge of Ghanaian college students relative to the disabled in Ghana. *Applied Research in Mental Retardation, 3,* 163-174.
Walker, S. (1983a). A comparison of attitudes personnel training needs and priorities relative to the disabled in Ghana and Nigeria. In K. Marfo, S. Walker & B. Charles (Eds.), *Education and rehabilitation of the disabled in Africa, Vol. 1: Towards improved services.* Edmonton: University of Alberta Center for International Education and Development.
Walker, S. (1983b). A comparison of personnel training needs and program priorities relative to the disabled in Ghana and Nigeria. *Journal of Negro Education, 52,* 162-166.

17

ATTITUDES TOWARD THE MENTALLY RETARDED: RESULTS FROM SIX COUNTRIES

A. Thomas Bickford & Edcil R. Wickham[1]

In recent years there have been remarkable changes in the prevention and amelioration of mental retardation (Clarke & Clarke, 1977; Sloan & Stevens, 1976). The implementation of laws promoting the concept of societal integration of the handicapped (e.g. Public Law 94-142 in the United States; the Development Services Act, 1974 in Ontario, Canada; and proposed Educational Bill 82 in Ontario, Canada) have spurred the development of new programs. Several authors have examined the concept of normalization and program evaluation (Schalock, Harper & Genung, 1981—USA; Keith, 1979—USA; Parham, 1979—USA; Skelton & Greenland, 1979—Canada; Wolfensberger, 1972—Canada, Sweden, USA); however, the success of these programs depends upon community acceptance and not just legislation and program planning.

The results of attempts to ascertain the public's opinion and acceptance of the mentally handicapped have been conflicting. A 1975 Gallup poll in the USA sponsored by the President's Committee on Mental Retardation (1976) showed respondents to be favorably disposed towards the mentally handicapped. However, the research of other Americans, namely, Gottlieb and his associates (Corman & Gottlieb, 1978; Gottlieb, 1975; Gottlieb & Corman, 1975; Gottlieb & Gottlieb, 1977; Gottlieb & Siperstein, 1976) has revealed mostly negative attitudes toward the mentally handicapped. Recent studies in Canada (Skelton & Greenland, 1979; Wilms, 1979); the United States (Kastner, Reppucci, & Pezzolli, 1979), and Britain (Furnham &

---

[1]This chapter is adapted from a paper presented at the 6th Congress of the International Association for the Study of Mental Deficiency, Toronto, August, 1982.

[2]The authors wish to acknowledge the Research Office of Wilfrid Laurier University for financial support and Audrey Leeman for her assistance in preparing the manuscript

Pendred, 1983) continue to yield examples of prejudice and negative attitudes toward this special population.

A basic tenet of normalization and mainstreaming is that contact with the retarded person or disabled individual would serve to dispel myths and false stereotypes. Gottlieb (1975) describes how a tour of an institution for the mentally retarded affected the attitudes of persons on the tour. The people's attitudes toward the staff of the institution improved while those toward the retarded persons declined. Corman and Gottlieb's (1978) review of research shows the controversy in the literature concerning public sentiment toward, and the success of contact with retarded persons. Recently Stager and Young (1981) found mixed benefits in the mainstreaming of retarded adolescents. These adolescents had better self-images than non-mainstreamed mentally retarded (MR) students. However, there was no increase in social interaction between MR students and their non-handicapped peers. Esposito and Peach (1983) also found an increase in handicapped children's self-concept and also noted an attitude change in the non-handicapped children.

In a slightly different context Gottlieb and Corman (1975) found that those respondents having no contact with retarded persons were more likely to favor segregation of retarded persons in the community. Jordan (1971) observed that it was not the contact alone that is related to attitudes, rather it is the quality and enjoyment of the contact which is most significantly related to attitudes. Gottlieb posits that "the more likely people are to believe that retarded people have a limited prognosis and should be segregated, the greater will be their beliefs that institutions are necessary to achieve these ends" (1975, p. 108). It is not surprising then that Sigelman and associates (Sigelman, 1976; Sigelman, Spanhe, & Lorensen, 1979) are cautious about enlisting the community's assistance during the planning stages. She reports that the greater the attempt to involve the community, the greater the number of objections and the louder the outcry against integration of the handicapped. Butterfield (1983) found that the strongest predictor of acceptance of an established group home was the extent of contact neighbors had with the residents.

The knowledge and attitudes of the professionals implementing the programs have also been examined. Contrary to expected beliefs, many helping agents are uninformed and/or have negative attitudes toward the mentally retarded (USA: Chubon, 1982; Jensema & Shears, 1971; Canada and USA: Morgan & Fevens, 1981).

Research on the underlying factors that comprise and predict public attitudes toward the mentally retarded has identified several factors. Social contact was found to be one of the main factors affecting attitudes (Voeltz, 1980; Kastner et al., 1979). Jordan (1971) reports four classes of variables: 1) econo-demographic factors (age, sex, income); 2) contact factors (amount, nature, enjoyment and perceived voluntariness; 3) socio-psychological factors (value orientation); and, 4) knowledge factors (the amount of factual information that would predict attitudes. Efron and Efron (1967) identified six factors within their study. These factors were: Segregation via Institutionalization (S/I); Cultural Deprivation; Non-contaminatory; Personal Exclusion (PE); Authoritarianism, and Hopelessness. Not much, however is presented on the study of these factors cross-culturally.

What little cross-cultural study that has been done is contradictory. Lippman (1974) discovered cultural differences between Europeans and North Americans. He observed three themes among Europeans: 1) a respect for dignity of the individual; 2) a genuine conviction that the mentally handicapped can be helped; and, 3) that there was an acceptance of social responsibility to help the handicapped. Stein and Susser (1980) found that in Southeast Asia the responsibility for MR persons rested with the family. This is the opposite of the European perception. Jordan (1971) posits that the underlying determinants would be culturally invariate. Our preliminary research is an attempt to measure some of these factors cross-culturally.

The *a priori* factors we considered to be important were: 1) Knowledge of Mental Retardation; 2) Social Contact (SC); 3) Social Responsibility (SR); 4) Educability of the Retarded (ER); and, 5) Employability (in the general work force). Even though Segregation by Institutionalization (S/I) is a major factor for Efron and Efron (1967), it was our hope to break down this factor into components. We expected to find demographic data which would separate groups based on age, sex, education, religion and social contact. We also expected to find differentiating characteristics among populations.

METHODOLOGY AND RESULTS

Questionnaires were administered in Barbados (n=455); Kenya (n=19); Peru (n=154); Prince Edward Island, Canada (n=140); Scotland (n=50); and Sierra Leone (n=22). Questionnaires having fewer than 80% of the questions answered were deleted. Communities sampled were not matched for this preliminary study and thus statistical comparisons cannot be made. Each sample will be commented on separately and trends among all populations will be presented.

The instrument used was presented in a 4-point Likert format requiring ratings from Agree (4) to Disagree (1). The neutral, undecided category was removed in order to force respondents to make an attitude preference.

Frequency distributions in percentages were obtained from each questionnaire. To compute a respondent's Total Acceptance of the Retarded score (TA) a score of 0 was assigned to Disagree, and a score of 3 to Agree. a high score indicated a pro-mentally retarded attitude and a low score suggested a negative or non-accepting attitude. The computed TA score was used as the dependent measure in separate analyses of variance with age, sex, education, occupation, religion and knowledge of a retarded person. To verify the attitudinal constructs (the *a priori* scales: knowledge, social contact, social responsibility, educability, and employability), the responses to the 20-item questionnaires were factor analyzed. The method used was the principal component analysis with iterations using a varimax orthogonal rotation (Kim, 1975).

BARBADOS

A majority of the respondents (80%) expressed accepting attitudes toward mentally retarded persons. The results indicate that younger people (age: $F_2=3.716$; $p<.05$), women (sex: $F_1=6.003$; $p<.02$), and those with less education (education: $F_4=4.714$; $p<.01$) were significantly more accepting of the retarded person. Subsequent Scheffe range tests indicated that specific subsets accounted for the variance. People having secondary school education were more disposed toward the retarded than university graduates, but there were no differences among other groupings. Similarly, the differences in the age groups were significant only between the "under 30" and the "30 to 40" age groups.

Table 1. A Comparison of Demographic Data Among Six Countries

BARBADOS	Sample	%	Age	%	Education	%	Religion	%	Occupation	%	Contact With M-R	%
	N = 445		Under 30	53.0	Primary	27.4	None	46.0	Unskilled	30.8	Some	67.8
	Women 202	45.4	30 - 40	26.0	Secondary	63.0	Protestant	25.5	Skilled	52.8	None	32.2
	Men 243	54.6	Over 40	21.0	University	9.6	Other	27.5	Professional	16.4		
KENYA	Sample	%	Age	%	Education	%	Religion	%	Occupation	%	Contact With M-R	%
	N = 19		Under 30	40.0	Primary		None	5	Unskilled	15.0	Some	75.0
	Women 13	65.0	30 - 40	15.0	Secondary	50.00	Protestant	25.0	Skilled	30.0	None	25.0
	Men 17	30.0	Over 40	45.0	University	50.00	Other	70.0	Professional	55.0		
PERU	Sample	%	Age	%	Education	%	Religion	%	Occupation	%	Contact With M-R	%
	N = 154		Under 30	31.8	Primary	3.9	None	2.0	Unskilled	26.0	Some	76.6
	Women 118	76.6	30 - 40	40.9	Secondary	38.0	R. Catholic	94.2	Skilled	11.7	None	23.4
	Men 36	23.4	Over 40	27.3	University	58.1	Other	3.8	Professional	62.3		
PRINCE EDWARD ISLAND	Sample	%	Age	%	Education	%	Religion	%	Occupation	%	Contact With M-R	%
	N = 140		Under 30	76.4	Primary	2.1	None	70.0	Unskilled	13.5	Some	75.0
	Women 69	49.3	30 - 40	7.9	Secondary	20.0	Protestant	18.5	Skilled	10.5	None	25.0
	Men 71	50.7	Over 40	15.7	University	77.9	Other	11.5	Professional	76.0		
SCOTLAND	Sample	%	Age	%	Education	%	Religion	%	Occupation	%	Contact With M-R	%
	N = 50		Under 30	16.0	Primary	4.0	None	16.0	Unskilled	36.0	Some	46.0
	Women 24	48.0	30 - 40	18.0	Secondary	62.0	Protestant	66.0	Skilled	38.0	None	54.0
	Men 26	52.0	Over 40	66.0	University	34.0	Other	18.0	Professional	26.0		
SIERRA LEONE	Sample	%	Age	%	Education	%	Religion	%	Occupation	%	Contact With M-R	%
	N = 22		Under 30	45.5	Primary	4.5	None	4.5	Unskilled	9.1	Some	72.7
	Women 5	22.7	30 - 40	27.3	Secondary	36.4	Protestant	77.3	Skilled	36.4	None	27.3
	Men 17	77.3	Over 40	27.3	University	59.1	Other	18.2	Professional	54.5		

The factor analysis yielded several factors with the first four accounting for 75% of the variance. Questions loading on the first factor suggested an S/I factor. The second loaded on questions indicating societal responsibility while the fourth showed a personal or non-societal responsibility. The factors were used as dependent measures with the demographic data in analysis of variance. The subsequent Sheffe range tests indicated similar results as with the TA scores, that is: the younger people, usually women, with less education and unskilled jobs were more disposed to the retarded.

KENYA

The sample was very supportive of the mentally retarded. Due to the small sample size the analysis of variance and factor analysis were not performed. It appears that in this sample to support the retarded may in part be due to the respondent having contact with a mentally retarded person.

PERU

The TA scores showed those sampled to be supportive (80%) of the retarded. The only significant result was with education ($F_3=3.629$; $p<.02$). Subsequent Sheffe range tests revealed that the differences existed only between post-graduate and primary schooling respondents, those with more education being more favorable of the retarded. The main factor to emerge was the S/I factor. The analysis of variance with the factors and the demographic data yielded no significant results. It must be noted that the sample population seemed highly skewed in favor of women and the data may not be representative of the general population.

PRINCE EDWARD ISLAND, CANADA

The respondents in this sample were far more positive (93%) than the other samples. The population had a large "under 30" component which may account for the high TA scores. The analysis indicated that women (sex: $F_1=5.07$; $p<.01$), and those having a religion other than Protestant (religion: $F_2=5.07$, $p<.01$) and people knowing a retarded person (personal knowledge: $F_1=5.725$, $p<.02$) were more supportive. The number one factor (52% of variance) loaded on social responsibility questions. The S/I factor was third for this population. When these factors were used in an analysis of variance the same demographic data were significant (sex, knowledge of retarded, and religion).

SCOTLAND

The population was generally supportive (79%) as well. The demographic data that yielded significant results were age (F_2=3.057, p<.05), education (F_3=4.325, p<.005, and religion (F_2=12.61, p<.001). These results indicate that younger persons, those with more education, and persons with a religion other than Protestant, were significantly more supportive of the retarded. The Sheffe range tests indicated that the only differences in attitude were between those having a university education and those with primary schooling only. The first factor (48% of variance) suggested the S/I factor. The second and third factor accounting for 28% of the variance loaded on the knowledge and social responsibility factors, respectively. A further analysis using the factors yielded only one significant main effect (SR and age: F_2= 4.019; p<.02).

SIERRA LEONE

The sample comprised a very high professional component which was supportive of the mentally retarded. Since this sample size was small, no analysis of variance or factor analysis was conducted. It appears that contact with the mentally retarded may account for this finding (72%).

IMPLICATIONS AND CONCLUSIONS

While statistical comparisons of the countries are not possible, the preliminary results indicate similarities across samples. The factor analysis produced three factors that appear to occur in each sample, namely, segregation and institutionalization, social responsibility and causes of retardation or basic knowledge. When these factors and the Total Acceptance scores were used as the dependent measures, there was an indication of support for the use of economic and demographic variables as predictors of public attitudes (Jordan, 1971). The general finding was that young people under age 30, women, and those having a higher education, appeared to have more positive attitudes towards the retarded. Only in the Prince Edward Island, Canada sample was personal contact with the retarded a predictor. There was an anomaly in the Scottish data indicating that less educated persons seemed to have more positive attitudes. This may have reflected a class difference, that the upper-class-people might have thought 'that one should take care of one's own, rather than an ignorance factor.

The common factor accounting for most of the variance in the samples was that of segregation and institutionalization. This supports Efron and Efron's (1967) findings among professionals of an underlying variable. There is also support for Jordan's (1971) hypothesis that the underlying determinant would be culturally invariant. The only sample that did not have the S/I factor as number one was that of Prince Edward Island, Canada. In that case the S/I factor was the third most important, accounting for 10% of the variance. This difference might be explained by the skewing of the sample in the young university-educated direction. This skewing may also account for the Social Responsibility factor ranking so highly (52% of the variance) as compared to other countries (10% or less of the variance).

The second most common factor was the Causes of Retardation or Basic Knowledge of Retardation factor. This may indicate a cognitive component in attitudes which would suggest that public education may help to change attidudes. However, as several authors have pointed out (Gottlieb & Gottlieb, 1977; Ajzen & Fishbein, 1977), attitudes do not reflect the person's behavioral intentions. Hence, the social planner must be concerned with education in the widest sense that emphasizes positive behavior towards the mentally handicapped person and is not limited to the cognitive aspect of attitudes.

These preliminary results must be cautiously examined. The large number of positive responses suggest that social desirability factors and questionnaire-demand characteristics need to be better controlled. In addition, the use of a broader base of questions, perhaps incorporating a behavioral component, is indicated. Future samples should be matched and more attention paid to sampling procedures, thus allowing for direct comparisons among countries.

The results of this study suggest that cross-cultural research may play a critical role in the determination of the underlying attitude variables. There is some indication that the econo-demographic variables of age, sex and level of education may be predictors of attitude response. Finally, the emergence of the three factors, Segregation/Institutionalization, Social Responsibility, and Knowledge support the notion of underlying variables. This may give program planners some direction as to the types of educational compaigns that could be implemented for the benefit of mentally handicapped persons.

References

Ajzen, I. & Fishbein, M. (1977). Attitude-behavior relations: A theoretical analysis and review of empirical research. *Psychological Bulletin, 84*, 888-918.

Butterfield, D. I. (1983). *Neighbor's perception of outdoor spaces surrounding group homes for the developmentally delayed adult.* Environmental Design Research Association.

Chubon, R. (1982). An analysis of research dealing with the attitudes of professionals toward disability. *Journal of Rehabilitation, 48*(1), 25-30.

Clarke, A. D. B. & Clarke, A. M. (1977). Prospects for prevention and amelioration of mental retardation: A guest editorial. *American Journal of Mental Deficiency, 81*, 523-533.

Corman, L. & Gottlieb, J. (1978). Mainstreaming mentally retarded children: A review of research. In N. Ellis (Ed.), *International Review of Research in Mental Retardation: Vol. 9*. New York: Academic Press.

Efron, R. E. & Efron, H. Y. (1967). Measurements of attitudes toward the retarded and an application with educators. *American Journal of Mental Deficiency, 72*, 100-107.

Esposito, B. G. & Peach, W. J. (1983). Changing attitudes of preschool children toward handicapped persons. *Exceptional Children, 49*, 361-363.

Furnham, A. & Pendred, J. (1983). Attitudes toward the mentally and physically disabled. *British Journal of Medical Psychology, 56*, 179-187.

Gottlieb, J. (1975). Public, peer, and professional attitudes toward mentally retarded persons. In M. J. Begab & S. A. Richardson (Eds.), *The mentally retarded and society: A social science perspective.* Baltimore: University Park Press.

Gottlieb, J. & Corman, L. (1975). Public attitudes toward mentally retarded children. *American Journal of Mental Deficiency, 80*, 72-80.

Gottlieb, J. & Gottlieb, B. W. (1977). Stereotypic attitudes and behavioral intentions toward handicapped children. *American Journal of Mental Deficiency, 82*, 65-72.

Gottlieb, J. & Siperstein, G. M. (1976). Attitudes toward mentally retarded persons: Effects of attitude referent specificity. *American Journal of Mental Deficiency, 80*, 376-381.

Jensema, C. J. & Shears, L. M. (1971). Attitudes of psychiatric technician trainees. *American Journal of Mental Deficiency, 76*, 170-175.

Jordan, J. E. (1971). Construction of a Guttman facet designed cross-cultural attitude-behavior scale toward mental retardation. *American Journal of Mental Deficiency, 76*, 201-219.

Kastner, L. S., Reppucci, N. D., & Pezzolli, J. J. (1979). Assessing community attitudes toward mentally retarded persons. *American Journal of Mental Deficiency, 84*, 137-144.

Keith, K. D. (1979). Behavior analysis: The principle of normalization. *AAESPH Review, 4*, 148-151.

Kim, J. O. (1975). Factor analysis. In N. Nie, C. H. Hull, J. G. Jenkins, K. Steinbrenner, & D. Bent (Eds.), *Statistical package for the social sciences: SPSS* (2nd Ed.). Toronton: McGraw Hill.

Lippman, L. D. (1974). *Attitudes toward the handicapped: A comparison between Europe and the United States.* Springfield, Ill.: C.C. Thomas.

Morgan, R. & Fevens, S. (1981). Transcending the iatrogenic approach to treating mentally retarded and learning disabled persons. *Psychological Reports, 49*, 47-54.

Parham, J. D. (1979). Developing an integrated community based system of extended rehabilitation services. *Journal of Rehabilitation, 75*, 64-67, 89.

President's Committee on Mental Retardation. (1976). *Mental retardation: Century of discussion.* Washington, D.C.: Department of Health, Education and Welfare (Publication No. OHD 76-21013.

Schalock, R., Harper, R., & Genung, T. (1981). Community integration of mentally retarded adults: Community placement program success. *American Journal of Mental Deficiency, 85*, 478-488.

Sigelman, C. K. (1976). A Machiavelli for planner: Community attitudes and selection for a group home site. *Mental Retardation, 14*(1), 15-20.

Sigelman, C. K., Spanhe, C. L., & Lorensen, C. D. (1979). Community reactions to deinstitutionalization: Crime, property values, and other bugbears. *Deficence Mentale/Mental Retardation, 29*(4), 15-20.

Skelton, M. & Greenland, C. (1979). Social work and mental retardation. In M. Craft (Ed.), *Tredgold's Mental Retardation* (12th Ed.). London: Baillière Tindall.

Sloan, W. & Stevens, H. A. (1976). *A century of concern: A history of the American Association on Mental Deficiency.* Washington, D.C.: American Association on Mental Deficiency.

Stager, S. F. & Young, R. D. (1981). Intergroup contact and social outcomes for mainstreamed EMR adolescents. *American Journal of Mental Deficiency, 85*, 497-507.

Stein, Z. & Susser, M. (1980). The less developed world: Souteast Asia as a paradigm. In J. Wortis (Ed.), *Mental Retardation and Developmental Disabilities: Annual Review* (XI). New York: Brunner/Mazel.

Voeltz, L. M. (1980). Children's attitudes toward handicapped peers. *American Journal of Mental Deficiency, 84*, 455-464.

Wilms, D. (1979). An investigation of public attitudes and concerns. *Mental Retardation, 29*(4), 10-15.

Wolfensberger, W. (1972). *The principle of normalization in human services.* Toronto: Leornard Crainford.

AUTHOR INDEX

T

U, V

W

Y, Z

SUBJECT INDEX

R, S, T

ABOUT THE EDITORS AND CONTRIBUTORS

THE EDITORS

KOFI MARFO is Assistant Professor of Special Education and Educational Psychology at Memorial University of Newfoundland, Canada. He has previously taught in elementary and secondary school settings and at the University of Cape Coast in Ghana. He has held a post-doctoral fellowship position at the University of Alberta where he was, until recently, Coordinator of the Cognitive Education Project directed by Dr. Robert Mulcahy. Dr. Marfo has published extensively on: early intervention; mother-child interaction processes involving mentally handicapped infants and young children; and education and rehabilitation of the disabled in developing countries. In addition to several book chapters and mimeographed books, he has published articles in a number of British and North American Journals: *Applied Research in Mental Retardation, Educational Psychology, Journal of Applied Developmental Psychology, Journal of Pediatric Psychology,* and *Mental Retardation (Toronto).* He is also co-editor, with Sylvia Walker and Bernard Charles, of *Education and rehabilitation of the disabled in Africa: Towards improved services* published in 1983 by the University of Alberta Center for International Education and Development. Dr. Marfo received his B.Ed. degree from the University of Cape Coast, Ghana, and his M.Ed. and Ph.D. degrees from the University of Alberta, Canada.

SYLVIA WALKER is Associate Professor in the School of Education and Graduate School of Arts and Sciences, Howard University, Washington, D.C. She is also Chairman of the Department of Psychoeducational Studies and Director of the Center for the Study of Handicapped Children and Youth at the School of Education. In addition to serving as a classroom teacher and administrator in several educational programs, she has participated in a number of teacher training, research, and service programs in the United States, South America, and Africa. She is currently providing leadership to a number of special projects, including the Howard University Model to Improve Rehabilitation Services to Minority Populations with Handicapping Conditions and the Competency Based Training Program to Prepare Teachers of the Severely Handicapped. Dr. Walker's publications have appeared in *Applied Research in Mental Retardation, the International Journal of Rehabilitation Research,* and *the Journal of Negro Education.* She has a B.A. degree from Queen's College, New York, an M.S. from Hunter College, New York, and M.Ed. and Ed.D. from Teachers College, Columbia University.

BERNARD CHARLES is a Program Officer for Carnegie Corporation of New York responsible for programs in: education, science, technology and the economy; prevention of damage to children (with emphasis on school failures); and human resources in developing countries. He was formerly Dean of Academic Affairs and Professor and Chairman of the Department of Urban Teacher Education at Livingston College, Rutgers University, New Jersey. He has been a guest lecturer at Fordham University, Columbia University, Yeshiva University, and the University of Cape Coast in Ghana. Mr. Charles is currently Vice President of the World Rehabilitation Fund, Chairman of the Board of the Public Education Association of New York City, member of the Boards of Trustees of Beth Israel Medical Center and Marymount College, and member of the Board of Directors of the Foundation for Children with Learning Disabilities. He has travelled extensively in Africa, the Caribbean, and Central and South America in connection with educational, rehabilitation, and human resource development programs. A graduate of Fisk University, Mr. Charles has a master's degree from Yeshiva University and has done advanced graduate studies at Columbia and Rutgers.

CONTRIBUTORS

BONIFACE J. AIDOO, M.Ed., is Lecturer in Human Development and Special Education at the University of Cape Coast, Ghana. He is currently completing his doctoral studies at George Peabody College, Vanderbilt University, Nashville, Tennessee.

ELIZABETH T. I. AKPATI, Ph.D., is Assistant Professor, Department of Communication Arts and Sciences, Howard University, Washington, D.C.

MARIA DA GRAÇA DE CAMPOS ANDRADA, M.D., is Consultant and Clinical Director at the Centro de Reabilitaçao de Paralisia Cerebral Calouste in Lisbon, Portugal. She is also the Director of the Pediatric Rehabilitation Service at the Centro de Medecina de Reabilitaçao, Alcoitao- Estoril, Portugal.

DAVID BAINE, Ed.D., is Professor of Special Education and Coordinator of the Multiple Dependent Handicapped Program in the Department of Educational Psychology, University of Alberta, Edmonton, Canada.

A. THOMAS BICKFORD, M.S.W., is affiliated with the Department of Family and Children's Services, Waterloo Region, Ontario, Canada. He is Supervisor at a residential facility for mentally handicapped adults.

MARG CSAPO, Ph.D., is Professor of Educational Psychology and Special Education, University of British Columbia, Vancouver, Canada. Dr. Csapo is Editor of the B. C. Journal of Special Education.

SAMUEL A. DANQUAH, Ph.D., is Professor and Research Consultant, Health Sciences Center-Faculty of Medicine, Memorial University of Newfoundland, St. John's, Canada.

TOM FRYERS, M.D., Ph.D., is Senior Lecturer in Community Medicine, University of Manchester, England, and Regional Specialist in Community Medicine, North West Regional Health Authority.

JOHN M. HUGHES, Ph.D., is Senior Lecturer, School of Special Education, Gwent College of Higher Education, Gwent, Wales.

M. MILES is Administrator of the Mental Health Center, Peshawar, North West Frontier Province, Pakistan. He is also Project Consultant to the FAMH/UNICEF Community Rehabilitation Development Project and General Secretary of the Society for Integrated Education of Handicapped Children.

FARHAT RASHID, B.Sc., is in charge of the Physiotherapy Department, Mental Health Center, Peshawar, Pakistan. She is also physiotherapy trainer for the FAMH/UNICEF Community Rehabilitation Development Project in the North West Frontier Province of Pakistan.

THE LATE G. ALLAN ROEHER, Ph.D., was Professor at York University, Toronto, Canada, a former President of the International Association for the Scientific Study of Mental Deficiency (IASSMD), and a former Director of the National Institute on Mental Retardation (NIMR), Canada.

MARIGOLD J. THORBURN, M.D., is Director of the Jamaica Early Stimulation Project and Regional Coordinator, Northern Technical Unit of the Caribbean Association on Mental Retardation and other Developmental Disabilities. She is also part-time Lecturer in the Pathology Department, University of the West Indies.

EDCIL R. WICKHAM, M.S.W., is Associate Professor, Faculty of Social Work, Wilfrid Laurier University, Waterloo, Ontario, Canada.

SULTANA S. ZAMAN, Ph.D., is Associate Professor of Psychology, Dhaka University, Bangladesh and Founder and General Secretary of the Bangladesh Protibondhi Foundation (Foundation for the Developmentally Disabled).